OXYGEN FIRST AID
for divers

Published by **J.L. Publications**
P.O. Box 381, Carnegie, Victoria 3163, Australia.
Telephone/Facsimilie: 61-3-569 4803

Australian edition published August 1992.
United States edition published December 1992.
United States edition reprinted with some alterations in 1995.
United Kingdom edition published 1994.

ISBN 0 9590306 5 4

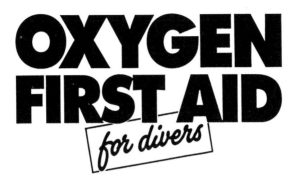

John Lippmann

United States Edition

J.L. Publications 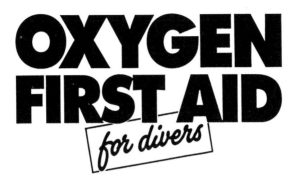 Melbourne

Preface

As long ago as 1878, Paul Bert demonstrated that oxygen breathing at one atmosphere relieved symptoms of cardiopulmonary decompression sickness in animals. Since then, a plethora of reports has confirmed these early findings and the breathing of 100% oxygen has now been firmly established as the first aid treatment of choice for decompression illness and certain other diving-related maladies.

Unfortunately, most divers, including divemasters and instructors, do not yet have the appropriate training to administer oxygen to divers who require it. However, the Divers Alert Network, and certain other organizations, have now established excellent courses designed to train divers in oxygen provision so that they can optimize the assistance given to a fellow diver in the event of a diving accident. This book has been written to be used as a text and/or further reference for such oxygen administration courses.

DISCLAIMER

There are some serious potential hazards associated with oxygen administration. Consequently, oxygen should not be administered by anyone untrained in its use. This book has been written to be used in conjunction with resuscitation and oxygen administration courses to supplement the information provided during the courses. *The book must not be used as a substitute for such training courses and the associated practice.*

This book represents the author's view of procedures for first aid resuscitation and oxygen administration to divers as at December 1992. However, the reader is warned that, while great care and effort has gone into the research for and preparation of this book, neither the author nor publisher warrants that the contents of this work will be entirely suitable for all circumstances which the reader may encounter. All potential oxygen providers should ensure that they are aware of and familiar with any local protocols, procedures, regulations or laws pertaining to resuscitation or oxygen administration.

It is stressed that first aid procedures vary from time to time and should never be used or adopted to the exclusion of, or in substitution for, medical consultation. The author and publisher make no claim that the information, practices and procedures given in this book will guarantee proper or adequate diagnosis and treatment of an individual who may or may not require pre-hospital oxygen administration.

Foreword

The on scene management of diving emergencies by providing oxygen first aid is an area of critical importance for all divers. An ever increasing body of evidence indicates that following the primary assessment (the ABC's), emergency oxygen is the single most effective first aid measure for decompression sickness (DCS), arterial gas embolism (AGE) and near drowning. In the most recent statistics from the Divers Alert Network (DAN), only 37 percent of injured divers received emergency oxygen at the scene, and few of those received anything approaching the recommended 100 percent. International diver training agencies and physicians familiar with diving medicine recommend the practice of providing 100 percent oxygen at the earliest possible moment once symptoms of a dive accident are recognized.

Statistics indicate that, under ideal conditions, metropolitan emergency medical services (EMS) response time is, on the average, 10 to 12 minutes for land-based emergencies. Enthusiastic divers, who search for the remote dive site where no one has gone before, further affect the prompt availability of emergency assistance, resulting in treatment delays of many hours or days. Prompt recognition of a diving-related emergency, and pre-EMS oxygen first aid for injured divers provided by trained and qualified personnel, may relieve signs and symptoms and enhance the results of hyperbaric treatment. It may reduce the likelihood of a permanent, debilitating injury, or be the difference between life and death.

The diving community is so convinced of the benefit of emergency oxygen first aid that some diver training agencies are currently recommending it as part of the annual scuba instructor renewal. Not providing emergency oxygen first aid falls short of accepted first aid guidelines and does not meet the first aid standard of practice for injured scuba divers.

Fundamental to any training program is a comprehensive textbook. This new book by John Lippmann, **Oxygen First Aid for Divers**, provides a resource of information unequaled. It encompasses a wide range of information, delivery equipment, and techniques satisfying the interests of the general diving public and the diving medical professional. All aspects of oxygen administration are presented in a concise and highly readable manner, including some unique techniques and philosophies. Written in a style which is easily comprehensible, it will serve as a valuable resource to diving and medical professionals alike.

Oxygen First Aid for Divers is thoroughly recommended to all who may be called upon to provide for the emergency needs of injured scuba divers using oxygen.

Dan Orr MS
Director of Training
Divers Alert Network

Peter B. Bennett PhD, DSc
Executive Director
Divers Alert Network

About the author

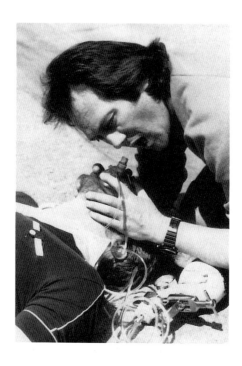

John Lippmann trained as a statistician and until recently was a mathematics lecturer at a College of Technical and Further Education in Melbourne, Australia. He has been an instructor and examiner in Oxygen Resuscitation and Sub-Aqua with the Royal Life-Saving Society of Australia (Vic.) for the past 12 years, being the Immediate Past Chairman of its Oxygen Resuscitation Panel and its representative on the Australian Resuscitation Council. He is also certified as a DAN Oxygen Intructor-Trainer with both DAN USA and DAN Australia.

John holds scuba instructor qualifications with a number of agencies and has specialized in teaching diver rescue, deep diving and oxygen administration courses. He has been responsible for the planning, coordinating and conducting of all Oxygen Resuscitation courses sanctioned by the Royal Life Saving Society of Australia (Vic.). Currently, as Executive Director and Director of Training of DAN Australia, John is responsible for the implementation and conduct of the DAN Australia Oxygen Programme.

John is the major author of **The DAN Emergency Handbook**, and the author of **Deeper Into Diving** and **The Essentials of Deeper Sport Diving**, all of which have gained worldwide recognition. He is also co-editor of **Scuba Safety in Australia**.

Acknowledgements

I wish to acknowledge the contributions of the editiorial panel and thank them sincerely for their constructive criticisms, contributions and support.

Members of the editorial panel were:

Dr. Chris Acott Coordinator DES/DAN Australia. Senior Specialist Anesthesiologist, Dept. of Anesthesia and Intensive Care; Senior Specialist, Hyperbaric Medicine Unit, Royal Adelaide Hospital, Adelaide, South Australia.

Dr. Peter Bennett Senior Director, F.G. Hall Hyperbaric Center. Executive Director, Divers Alert Network. Professor of Anesthesiology and Associate Professor of Neurobiology and Cell Biology, Duke University Medical Center, Durham, North Carolina.

Jeffrey Bertsch DMT-A, CHT. Training Specialist, Divers Alert Network, Durham, North Carolina.

James Corry Chairman of the Diving and Water Rescue Committee of the National Association for Search and Rescue. Program Director of the Water Safety Program of the U.S. Secret Service. American Red Cross CPR and First Aid Instructor. NAUI Instructor Trainer.

Surgeon Commander Des Gorman Director of Occupational, Diving and Hyperbaric Medicine, Royal New Zealand Naval Hospital. Senior Lecturer in Anesthesia and Intensive Care, University of Adelaide, South Australia. Current President, South Pacific Underwater Medicine Society (SPUMS).

Terry Grimmond Chief Scientist and Lecturer, Dept. of Microbiology and Infectious Diseases, Flinders Medical Center, South Australia.

Dr. John Knight Visiting Anesthesiologist, Royal Victorian Eye and Ear Hospital, Melbourne, Victoria, Australia. Current Editor, SPUMS Journal.

Dr. David Komesaroff A Senior Specialist Anesthesiologist, Royal Melbourne Hospital. Director of Anesthesia, Sandringham & District Memorial Hospital, Victoria, Australia. Ex-Chairman, Australian Resuscitation Council (Vic).

Dr. Bart McKenzie Specialist Anesthesiologist, Princess Alexandra Hospital, Brisbane. Ex-Officer-in-Charge, Royal Australian Navy School of Underwater Medicine, Sydney, Australia.

Dr. Giles Yancey Mebane Associate Medical Director, Divers Alert Network. Assistant Professor of Community and Family Medicine, Duke University Medical Center, Durham, North Carolina.

Dr. Richard Moon Associate Professor of Anesthesiology, Assistant Professor of Pulmonary Medicine, Duke University Medical Center, Durham, North Carolina. Medical Director, Duke Hyperbaric Center. Medical Director, Divers Alert Network.

Dan Orr Director of Training, Divers Alert Network, Durham, North Carolina.

Betty Orr Membership Coordinator, Divers Alert Network, Durham, North Carolina.

Dr. Harry Oxer Director of Hyperbaric Medicine, Fremantle Hospital, Western Australia. Ex-Chairman, Australian Resuscitation Council (Federal). Medical Director, St John Ambulance (WA).

David Reinhard Advanced Life Support Ambulance Officer, Metropolitan Ambulance Service, Victoria, Australia.

Dr. John Williamson Director, Hyperbaric Medicine Unit, Royal Adelaide Hospital, Adelaide, South Australia. Senior Lecturer in Anesthesia, University of Adelaide. National Deputy Director of Training, St John Ambulance. St John Ambulance representative on Australian Resuscitation Council. PADI Instructor Emeritus.

I wish to convey my special appreciation to Dan Orr and Jim Corry for the enormous support and encouragement they have given me in preparing this United States edition of my book. Jim's numerous articles on oxygen administration provided a lot of important information necessary to create this edition. I am grateful to Jim for his permission to reprint much of this information. I had the privilege and pleasure of attending a DAN Oxygen First Aid in Diving Accidents Course conducted by Dan Orr. He is a truly inspirational, informative and very humorous lecturer. I heartily encourage all divers to attend the DAN Oxygen Course.

I wish to acknowledge the contributions of Judge Tom Wodak (Diving Instructor and previously an Attorney at Law specializing in medico-legal litigation) and Michael Gatehouse (Diving Instructor and Attorney at Law involved in diving litigation), who co-authored the chapter on Legal Considerations with me, and James Page (Attorney at Law and Publisher, Journal of Emergency Medical Services (JEMS)) who checked its content and suitability for the United States; Frances Birrell (Infection Control Nurse, Fairfield Hospital, Melbourne) and Ella Tyler (Deputy Chairman, Australian Resuscitation Council) for editing the chapter on disease transmission. Thanks also to Larry "Harris" Taylor for supplying various data from his vast library, to Steve Neese for his technical advice and support.

Finally, I wish to express gratitude to my wife, Angela, and sons, Michael and Adam, for still not taking me seriously when I said I wouldn't write yet another book.

OXYGEN FIRST AID
for divers

- CONTENTS -

Page

Chapter 1

RESPIRATION AND CIRCULATION

THE RESPIRATORY SYSTEM

FIGURE 1.1
The respiratory system

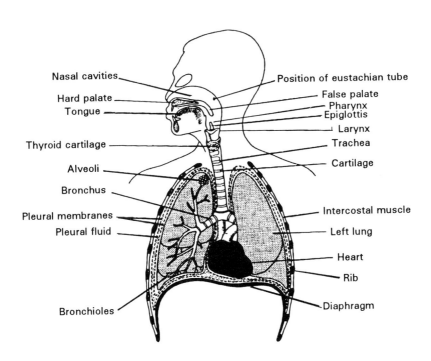

The respiratory tract extends from the opening of the mouth and nose to the tiny alveoli in the lungs.

Air is drawn into the mouth and nose and is warmed and humidified in these structures. The air passes through the *pharynx*, which is a short, common pathway for air and food. The pharynx divides into two tubes - the *trachea* (windpipe) and the *esophagus* (gullet). The esophagus lies behind the trachea and takes food and fluids into the stomach. Air travels through the *larynx* or voice box which is at the top of the trachea. Food is normally prevented from entering the larynx by reflex closure of the vocal cords during swallowing, assisted by a cartilaginous flap known as the *epiglottis*. After passing through the larynx, air enters the trachea, which contains a series of semi-circular rings of cartilage in front, and is closed behind by tissue. The trachea passes down into the chest where it divides into two main tubes; the right and left *bronchi*. One bronchus (singular for bronchi) goes to each lung. Inside the lungs, the bronchi divide into smaller tubes, called *bronchioles*, which are also supported by cartilage rings. The bronchioles also continue to divide until they end in air sacs, the *alveoli*, of which there are approximately 150 to 250 million in each adult lung. The trachea and bronchi are lined by cells covered with tiny hairs, *cilia*, which are kept moist by glands. The cilia move foreign particles up and away from the lungs.

The two lungs are cone-shaped and are situated in the chest. They are composed of elastic tissue and are protected by the breastbone or *sternum* in front, the spine from behind, and by the ribs. The first seven ribs of each side are attached directly to the sternum. The next three are attached to the ribs just above, while the front ends of the last two are free. The ribs, sternum and spine form the *thoracic cage*. Between the ribs lie the *intercostal muscles*, which participate in the action of breathing. The chest is closed below and is separated from the *abdomen* by the *diaphragm*, which is a dome-shaped muscle attached to the spine and lower ribs. The diaphragm is composed of muscle and strong fibrous tissue. The thoracic cage also protects the *heart* and the largest blood vessels.

FIGURE 1.2

The thoracic cage

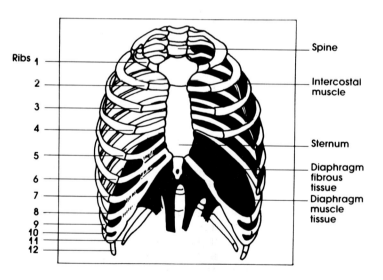

Each lung is surrounded by two layers of very thin membrane, the *pleura*. One layer covers the lung itself and the other the chest wall. The space enclosed between the pleura is called the *pleural cavity.* It is normally only a potential cavity since the two layers of pleura are held together by the surface tension of a thin layer of lubricant that facilitates movement.

MECHANISM OF BREATHING

During quiet, spontaneous breathing, the diagphragm descends, and in deeper breathing the combination of expansion of the chest wall plus diaphragm movement further increases the size of the chest cavity. As the lungs expand, the pressure of air in the expanded lungs becomes lower than that in the atmosphere, creating a pressure gradient and drawing air through the nose or mouth and into the lungs.

When the diaphragm relaxes, the chest cavity decreases in size. This raises the pressure in the lungs above ambient pressure and forces air from the lungs.

THE CIRCULATORY SYSTEM

The Heart

The heart is in the middle of the chest behind the sternum, and extends somewhat to the left side. It is a strong muscular pump, which in the average adult sends about six liters of blood through well over 1,000 complete circuits of the body each day. The heart consists of two independent but joined pump systems, one on the left side of the heart and one on the right side. The left pump is far more powerful than the right. Each pump has two chambers - the *atrium*, which receives blood from the body and lungs; and the *ventricle*, which is filled with blood from the atrium. The left ventricle pumps blood throughout the body and the right ventricle pumps blood to the lungs.

When the ventricles contract, blood cannot return to the atria because of one-way valves. Blood pumped out of the ventricles is also prevented from returning by valves.

When blood leaves the left ventricle, it passes up the *aorta*, which is the largest artery in the body. The aorta gives off a number of branches, which include the *carotid arteries* to the brain, and ends by dividing into arteries which supply blood to the lower limbs.

The arteries have thick, elastic walls that resist stretching, thereby maintaining the blood pressure by elastic recoil. Blood only flows through the arteries when it is pumped out by the heart. The swelling of an artery as blood passes down it is what we can feel over an artery, and is known as a *pulse*. The arteries become smaller as they divide into smaller *arterioles* and finally into the tiny *capillaries*, the smallest blood vessels. It is in the capillaries that *oxygen* and *carbon dioxide* exchange takes place. From capillaries, the blood is gathered into small, thin-walled veins and then into larger veins before finally returning to the right atrium of the heart. Most larger veins direct the blood flow by means of one-way valves which prevent the blood travelling in the wrong direction.

From the right atrium, the blood passes to the right ventricle to be pumped through the pulmonary arteries to the lungs. The pulmonary arteries are the only arteries containing relatively poorly oxygenated blood. In the lungs, the blood takes up oxygen, facilitates the removal of carbon dioxide, and returns to the left atrium through the pulmonary veins. Pulmonary veins are the only veins containing oxygenated blood.

The heart itself needs considerable oxygen to function adequately and has its own blood vessels, the *coronary arteries*, to supply its needs.

Composition of Blood

Blood is a fluid containing solid cells. The fluid part, known as the *plasma*, comprises about 55% of the blood. It carries sugar for energy, other nutritional compounds and various other substances including some dissolved oxygen. The cellular part of the blood consists of the following cell groups:

(1) The *red cells* (erythrocytes) are the most numerous and carry *hemoglobin* which bonds with oxygen and gives the blood its characteristic red color. When the blood is fully oxygenated it is bright red in color, but this color diminishes as the oxygen is used up.

(2) The *white cells* (leukocytes), which fight bacterial and viral infection.

(3) The *platelets*, which are the smallest of the blood cells. Platelets begin the process of blood clotting when a blood vessel is injured or a foreign body enters the bloodstream.

Oxygen

Oxygen is a colorless, odorless and tasteless gas that constitutes about 21% of the air we breathe. We need oxygen to effectively metabolize food and provide energy for cell function. The body consumes oxygen and produces carbon dioxide, as well as heat and other forms of energy.

The blood carries oxygen in two forms: chemically combined with hemoglobin and dissolved in plasma.

Since oxygen is not very soluble in plasma at normal temperatures and pressures, very little is normally dissolved in plasma. The vast majority of oxygen is chemically combined with hemoglobin. When breathing air at normal atmospheric pressures, the hemoglobin is 97.5% saturated with oxygen. As the oxygen rich blood reaches the tissues, the hemoglobin releases some oxygen to the tissues but still remains about 75% saturated.

Hypoxia

When our body tissues receive too little oxygen, they become hypoxic. *Hypoxia* is a state of low tissue oxygen levels, and *anoxia* is a complete lack of oxygen. The term *hypoxemia* is sometimes used to describe lower than normal oxygen levels in arterial blood.

Body cells cannot survive for long without oxygen. Brain cells and cells of the nervous system are particularly sensitive to hypoxia and can die in minutes (usually about four minutes for brain cells).

There are many ways that tissue hypoxia can occur. Airway obstruction or lung damage are common causes of hypoxemia, which leads to tissue hypoxia. Too little oxygen in the gas we breathe also results in hypoxemia. This will occur when the partial pressure of oxygen falls below about 0.16 atmospheres absolute (ATA). Poisoning with carbon monoxide interferes with oxygen transport by hemoglobin, and oxygen utilization in the tissues. Cyanide prevents the cells taking up oxygen by poisoning enzyme systems. Bubbles resulting from decompression illness may block or damage an arteriole, thereby cutting off the blood supply and causing hypoxia beyond the blockage by preventing the arrival of oxygen-carrying blood. The same happens when blood flow through a part of the body is reduced by constriction of arterioles, perhaps due to the effects of cold, or a fall in blood pressure.

Symptoms of hypoxia appear suddenly and progress rapidly. They include: Inability to recognize a decrement in performance; drowsiness; incoordination; headache; slurred speech; double vision; possible euphoria; apathy; blueness of lips, mouth and fingernail beds (*cyanosis*); rapid pulse and breathing; convulsions; unconsciousness and death. Prompt treatment is required to prevent permanent brain damage. First aid involves the establishment of an adequate airway, further resuscitation if required, and oxygen provision if oxygen equipment is available.

Carbon Dioxide

Carbon dioxide is a waste product of our metabolism. Most of it is carried in our blood as carbonic acid, which is a weak acid made from a chemical combination of carbon dioxide and water. As the carbon dioxide diffuses from the tissues into the blood, the acidity of the blood increases. This increased carbon dioxide is detected by acidity receptors in the brain, and the rate and depth of breathing is adjusted until the acidity is reduced to normal levels.

Hypercapnia

An excess of carbon dioxide in the blood is called *hypercapnia*. Hypercapnia can be caused by any interference with the process of carbon dioxide transport and elimination. If allowed to accumulate in the body, carbon dioxide will eventually exert a toxic effect. The signs and symptoms of carbon dioxide toxicity depend on the rate of build-up of the carbon dioxide and the amount of carbon dioxide present. The first sign is often an increase in the depth and rate of breathing. Shortness of breath with rapid, deep breathing occurs and may be followed by a throbbing headache. If the level continues to rise, dizziness, nausea, confusion, unsteadiness, disorientation and restlessness may result. The person may become flushed and their face may feel warm. Lightheadedness, muscle twitches and jerks, reduced vision, unconsciousness, tremors and convulsions may occur as the level continues to increase. Although death can occur in rare cases, recovery from carbon dioxide toxicity is usual.

Varying degrees of hypercapnia can arise during oxygen provision if the system is inadequately supplied with fresh gas, and the injured diver is allowed to rebreathe too much expired breath.

GAS EXCHANGE

The alveoli have extremely thin walls which are only one cell thick and are surrounded by a dense network of capillaries. They can be likened to tiny air spaces with the configuration of a very fine sponge. Only a tiny distance (roughly 1/20 of the thickness of this page) separates the gas in the alveoli from the blood in the capillary. The barrier between gas and blood is sometimes called the alveolar-capillary membrane. If this membrane is torn and alveolar air enters the blood, an air embolism results. However, the membrane does not necessarily need to be torn or damaged for air to enter the circulatory system. Air may actually be forced through the thin alveolar walls directly into the capillaries with no physical damage to lung tissue.

FIGURE 1.3

An alveolus surrounded by capillaries

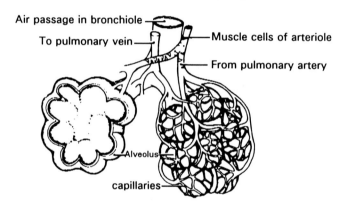

Air passage in bronchiole

To pulmonary vein

Muscle cells of arteriole

From pulmonary artery

Alveolus

capillaries

Reprinted with permission of P. Gadd and Macmillan Publishers Ltd.

It is across this alveolar-capillary membrane that the exchange of oxygen and carbon dioxide occurs. This passage of gas across the alveolar-capillary membrane is called *diffusion*. Diffusion is the passage of a gas from an area where it has a high concentration to an area of lower concentration, until the concentrations are equal. (Figure 1.4).

After inspiration, the concentration of oxygen in the alveoli is higher than in the blood in the lung capillaries. This causes oxygen to diffuse from the alveoli into the blood. Simultaneously, carbon dioxide diffuses from the blood, where its concentration is higher, into the lungs where its concentration is lower. Most of the carbon dioxide is then exhaled.

When the lungs expand during inspiration, the capillaries next to the alveoli are stretched out and "pulled open", resulting in an increase in blood flow (*perfusion*) through them. In addition, the area of contact between the alveoli and the surrounding capillaries is increased, producing ideal conditions for the transfer of gases between the alveoli and the blood in the capillaries.

If all the alveoli were opened out and laid flat, they would cover an area of about the size of a tennis court. This provides a large surface area for gas exchange.

FIGURE 1.4

Exchange of gases across the alveolar-capillary membrane

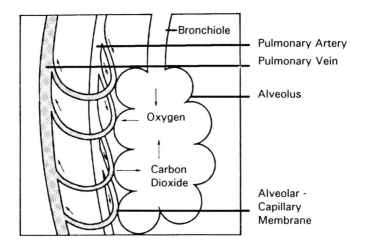

To ensure oxygen enters the blood, the oxygen supply must be constantly renewed. In order to achieve this, the air in the lungs must be constantly changed by breathing, which is sometimes called respiratory ventilation.

Breathing is essentially rhythmical, the rhythm is established shortly after birth and changes its rate with age, health and exertion.

CONTROL OF BREATHING

The partial pressure of carbon dioxide in the arterial blood is the dominant factor regulating breathing.

The *medulla,* which is the respiratory center located in the brain stem, contains groups of nerve cells, called *chemoreceptors.* These chemoreceptors are sensitive to acid (hydrogen ions). When blood laden with carbon dioxide reaches the brain, the medulla sends nerve impulses to the diaphragm and other respiratory muscles, making them contract and causing inspiration and the subsequent removal of carbon dioxide with expiration. The depth and frequency of breathing is adjusted so that carbon dioxide is discharged in the expired gas at the same rate as it is produced in the tissues. This ensures a continuous, even stimulus to breathe, producing regular inspiration and expiration.

Respiration stimulated by carbon dioxide also ensures that the oxygen intake from the lungs remains at a rate which satisfies the needs of the body.

Lack of oxygen does not normally stimulate breathing significantly unless the arterial oxygen levels fall dangerously low. Other chemoreceptors which are sensitive to low arterial oxygen are located in the walls of the aorta and the carotid arteries, and will stimulate the breathing if oxygen levels fall dramatically.

SOME PHYSIOLOGICAL DEFINITIONS AND NORMAL VALUES

Dead space: Dead space is that part of the respiratory tract that does not take part in gas exchange. The anatomical dead space is the nose, mouth, pharynx, trachea and larger bronchi. People with some chest conditions, such as emphysema, have increased dead space. Using a snorkel or regulator increases dead space significantly. Dead space is sometimes defined as the part of the tidal volume that does not participate in gas exchange. It is the gas that is in the airways rather than in the alveoli. In a normal person, it is around one third of the tidal volume.

Total lung capacity: This is the total volume of gas in the lungs. It averages approximately 6 liters in an adult.

Tidal volume: This is the volume of gas that moves in and out of the lungs with each breath. An average 150 pound adult has a tidal volume of around 500 ml while at rest.

Respiratory rate: This is the number of breaths per minute and is usually 12-15 breaths per minute for an adult.

Respiratory minute volume: The minute volume is defined as the amount of gas breathed in or out during one minute. It is the tidal volume multiplied by the respiratory rate, and is typically around 6 liters per minute for an adult at rest.

Pulse rate: Is generally 60-80 beats per minute in an adult but varies with age, health and fitness.

Oxygen consumption: This is the amount of oxygen consumed by the body's metabolism within one minute. It is approximately 250 ml per minute in an average adult at rest.

Carbon dioxide production: This is the amount of carbon dioxide produced by the body's metabolism within one minute. It is generally about 200 ml per minute in an average adult at rest.

REVIEW QUESTIONS

1. List the major differences between veins and arteries.
2. List the main constituents of blood and briefly describe their function.
3. How is oxygen transported through the body?
4. Briefly describe the process of diffusion.
5. What provides the main trigger to breathe?
6. List six signs or symptoms of hypoxia.
7. List six signs or symptoms of hypercapnia.
8. What is the average tidal volume of an adult at rest?

Chapter 2

CIRCULATORY FAILURE - SHOCK

Shock occurs when the circulation is inadequate to meet the oxygen demands of the major body organs. Essential organs such as the heart, brain, lungs and kidneys therefore receive less oxygen than they need to fully function.

The inadequate circulation may be due to an actual physical loss of blood from severe bleeding, whether external or internal, or loss of other body fluids due to excessive sweating, burns, diarrhea and vomiting. On the other hand, the inadequate circulation can result from a physiological loss where, although there is no actual blood loss, a redistribution of blood or a leaking of plasma into the tissues leads to the same overall response as if it were lost. For example, if blood is redirected to a specific area to fight a severe infection, less blood is available to supply oxygen to the brain and other vital organs. Decompression sickness can cause capillaries to leak fluid into the surrounding tissues, thereby reducing the volume of circulating blood.

Shock may result from any condition that decreases the heart's ability to pump effectively or decreases the return of blood from the veins to the heart. It can be associated with many different illnesses or injuries.

Regardless of the cause of shock, the effects are essentially the same. The body tries to compensate for the reduced circulation by: (1) reducing the blood supply to the skin, gut and kidneys and redirecting it to more vital areas. It achieves this by constricting the blood vessels to the non-essential areas; (2) increasing the breathing rate to increase the intake of oxygen; (3) increasing the heart rate to circulate the remaining blood more rapidly, thereby increasing oxygen delivery.

The signs and symptoms of shock are produced by the combination of the lack of oxygen supply to the tissues and the body's response to it.

The signs and symptoms of shock include cold, clammy, pale skin; rapid shallow breathing; a rapid, weak pulse; and nausea.

Probably the most obvious sign of shock is pale, clammy, cold skin. The reduced circulation to the skin causes it to be pale and cold, and nervous system stimulation of the sweat glands causes the clamminess. Breathing becomes rapid and shallow as the body tries to take in more oxygen. The heart rate is increased to circulate more oxygen, but, since the faster-beating heart cannot fill as effectively, and because of the reduced circulating blood volume, blood pressure is reduced. Hence, the pulse feels rapid and weak. Lack of oxygen to the brain may result in dizziness, confusion and a reduced level of consciousness. Other signs and symptoms include weakness, thirst, nausea, vomiting and apprehension.

The body can only compensate temporarily and, if the underlying cause is not treated or corrected, the diver may deteriorate rapidly. A diver who has suffered a substantial loss of blood or other body fluids will eventually deteriorate and become severely ill unless blood volume is restored.

First aid for shock includes the following steps:

- **Monitoring the airway, breathing and pulse.** Improvement can be seen by improvement in mental clarity, the pulse becoming stronger and slower, and the breathing slowing to a more normal rate and depth.
- **Determining the cause and acting to rectify it, if possible.** Severe external bleeding must be stopped immediately.
- **Laying the diver down.** Blood flow to the brain is improved by laying the injured diver flat with the legs raised. An unconscious (breathing) or nauseated diver should be placed in a stable side (recovery) position.
- **Providing oxygen.** Oxygenation of the body tissues is improved by increasing the concentration of inspired oxygen.
- **Arranging medical assistance or advice.** Many first aiders lack adequate experience to determine whether further treatment will be required. Appropriate medical advice should be sought. Remember that if the cause of shock is not rectified the diver may deteriorate rapidly.
- **Keeping the diver still, quiet and reassured.** The injured diver is kept still to minimize the blood flow to the muscles, thereby maximizing the supply to vital organs and allowing the body to stabilize. Anxiety increases the effects of shock, so the injured diver must be reassured.
- **Protecting the diver from hazards and extremes of temperature.** Shelter the diver from the elements and maintain a comfortable, near-normal body temperature. Overwarming causes opening up of peripheral blood vessels and leads blood away from where it is needed most.
- **Giving nothing by mouth.** Circulation to the stomach and intestines is reduced as the body compensates for shock. Giving the diver food or drinks may precipitate vomiting. In addition, if the diver later becomes unconscious or requires a general anesthetic, the likelihood of vomiting or regurgitation will be increased. However, in some circumstances it may be appropriate to give certain fluids, such as water. One such situation is when the shock is associated with decompression illness. Alcohol and sedatives must not be given as they depress central nervous system function. In addition alcohol causes dilation of peripheral blood vessels and counteracts the body's defences against shock. Stimulants such as coffee, tea or cigarettes should not be given as they speed up an already overworking, compensating body.
- **Keeping a clear record** of the circumstances and time of the accident, the changing state of the injured diver and any treatment given and how much blood/fluid (e.g. vomit) the injured diver has lost.

FIGURE 2.1
Injured diver being treated for shock

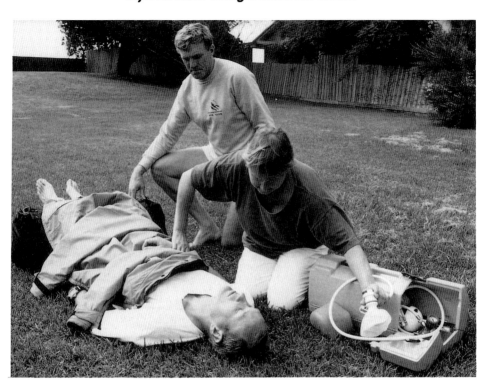

REVIEW QUESTIONS:

1. What is shock and how does the body attempt to compensate for it?
2. List 5 common signs or symptoms of shock.
3. Briefly summarize the steps in the first aid for shock.
4. Why is it important to seek medical aid when treating a diver for shock?

Chapter 3

RESUSCITATION

Resuscitation is the preservation or restoration of life by the establishment and/or maintenance of the Airway, Breathing and Circulation (ABC) and related emergency care.

Current resuscitation techniques are aimed at preserving life and, by maintaining an adequate supply of oxygen to the brain, preventing the irreversible brain damage which results if the brain is deprived of oxygen for more than a few minutes. Death of brain tissue usually commences after about 3-5 minutes of oxygen deprivation, depending on the age and general condition of the injured person, among other factors. **If resuscitation is required, it should be commenced immediately to maximize the injured diver's chances of recovery.**

The appropriate resuscitation technique depends upon the condition of the injured diver, the training and skill of the first aider, and the available equipment, if any. Techniques range from simply establishing a patent (clear and open) airway, to *rescue breathing* (sometimes called *expired air resuscitation*), *cardiopulmonary resuscitation* (CPR), the provision of oxygen and the use of defibrillators and/or drugs to restore normal heart action.

ASSESSMENT

It is extremely important to assess the condition of the injured diver carefully before commencing any resuscitative procedures, such as repositioning the diver, opening the airway and commencing rescue breathing.

On discovering the seemingly unconscious diver, the first aider must quickly assess any injury and determine whether the diver is in fact unconscious. If it is suspected that the diver may have sustained injury to the head and neck (neck injuries are uncommon in the diving situation), movement must be minimized to avoid aggravating the injury.

The first aider should speak to the diver (if on the surface) in a loud voice and ask if they are OK. Tapping or *gently* shaking the diver may elicit a response if they are conscious. Squeezing the injured diver's hand while asking them to squeeze your hand can sometimes prove useful in determining the level of consciousness.

These precautions may help prevent injury from the attempted resuscitation of a diver who does not require it, or assault of the would-be rescuer!

CALL FOR HELP

After assessing the level of consciousness, the next step is to activate the Emergency Medical Services (EMS).

Call for help from bystanders since they may be needed to activate the Emergency Medical Services (EMS) systems and to assist you in other ways.

It is a good idea to have an emergency assistance (or action) plan (EAP). The EAP includes vital emergency information, including how to activate or contact the local EMS or medical facility. The EAP can be written on the appropriate pages of **The DAN Emergency Handbook**, which is waterproof so that it can be kept with the dive gear and easily taken to the dive site.

EMS is activated by dialing the local emergency number (911, if available). Ensure that the person activating the EMS knows the relevant details of: (1) where the emergency is; (2) the telephone number from which the call is made; (3) the nature of the problem; (4) how many people need help; (5) the condition of the injured diver(s); and (6) what aid is being provided. The caller should hang up last to ensure the EMS personnel have no further questions.

The importance of getting appropriately trained medical help as soon as possible cannot be overstated. This is especially true if the diver's heart has stopped beating effectively, as discussed later.

When sending someone to activate the EMS, ensure that they know:

- who to contact and the appropriate emergency phone number(s)
- the location of the injured diver(s)
- how many injured divers
- the condition of the injured diver(s)

Ask the person who is going for help to repeat these details to you so that you can correct them if necessary. Also ask them to return to you immediately after they have summoned help. In this way you will know if the EMS has in fact been activated.

POSITION THE INJURED DIVER

If the injured diver has sustained injury to the head and neck, or if such an injury is suspected, the first aider should move the injured diver only if absolutely necessary. Improper movement may cause paralysis in the diver with a neck injury.

An unconscious diver who is breathing spontaneously should be placed in the *recovery position* (Figure 3.3) if no neck injury is suspected. Placement in the recovery position consists of rolling the injured diver onto the side to help protect the airway. Care must be taken to minimize bending and twisting (rotation) of the neck. The injured diver's entire body should be rolled over simultaneously.

For resuscitative efforts and evaluation to be effective, the injured diver must be supine and on a firm, flat surface. If it is necessary to roll the injured diver onto the back, it must be done carefully to minimize rotation of the neck, and the injured diver's entire body should be rolled over simultaneously. Once the diver is supine, the arms should be placed alongside the body.

A unconscious diver must be handled gently with no twisting or forward movement of the head and neck.

The ABC of resuscitation is then implemented as appropriate.

A - CHECK THE AIRWAY

RESPIRATORY FAILURE

Respiratory failure is said to occur when a person's breathing becomes inadequate or ceases. Depressed or absent breathing leads to inadequate oxygenation of the blood (hypoxemia) and, therefore, an insufficient supply of oxygen to the brain and other organs.

Respiratory failure commonly occurs because the airway is obstructed. In an unconscious person, the obstruction is usually caused by the relaxed tongue falling back and blocking the pharynx, or the presence of foreign matter such as water, vomitus, blood or some other foreign object in the upper airway. Foreign matter in the upper airways can cause spasm and closure of the larynx (called *laryngospasm*) which may last up to about two minutes. This is long enough for the person to become *cyanotic* (blue) from the lack of oxygen in the blood. Laryngospasm may recur if the problem is not rectified.

Complete airway obstruction is silent since there is no air flow. If it is not corrected quickly, breathing attempts will stop (*apnea*) and the heart will normally stop beating (*cardiac arrest*) within about 5 to 10 minutes. (However, this time may occasionally be extended for periods of up to 60 minutes in the case of cold water near drowning, especially in children). Partial airway obstruction is noisy since the air is trying to force itself through narrowed airways. If not promptly corrected, partial obstruction can also lead to serious hypoxemia and consequent tissue hypoxia.

AIRWAY MANAGEMENT

In a large number of cases, where breathing has stopped as a result of a blocked airway, simply providing an open airway will allow breathing to recommence as long as the heart is still beating.

If an unconscious person is left lying on the back, the lower jaw (*mandible*) drops back and the tongue, which is attached to the jaw, drops back against the back of the throat, thereby partly or completely blocking the passage of air to the lungs. The relaxation of the soft palate (roof of the mouth) and the epiglottis in the unconscious person may increase the blockage. Because an unconscious person loses the ability to swallow and cough, saliva and other foreign material can accumulate in the airway and aggravate the problem.

Fluid, blood or other visible foreign material can be scooped out by the first aider's fingers, but care should be taken not to insert the fingers too far or for too long as it may precipitate gagging or vomiting. Care should also be taken that the injured diver cannot bite or clench the teeth before the first aider inserts their fingers. Loose dentures should be removed as they may dislodge and block the airway. Secure dentures can usually be left in place as they help keep the airway open and facilitate a good seal when doing rescue breathing.

Head tilt and chin lift

If there is no evidence of head or neck injury, the first aider should use the *head tilt/chin lift maneuver* to open the airway. Tilting the injured diver's head back and supporting the jaw by lifting the chin should create an open airway. This is easily achieved by placing one hand on the diver's forehead while lifting the chin with the other hand. The head is then gently tilted with a fulcrum action. Care must be taken not to place your fingers on the soft tissues of the injured diver's neck since it may interfere with the airway or circulation to or from the brain.

FIGURE 3.1

Head tilt and chin lift

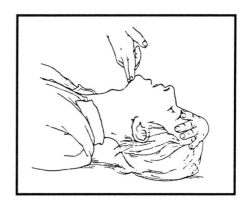

Head tilt and chin lift is simple, safe and easily learned, and is the method of choice in most basic resuscitation situations. However, an alternative technique, known as *jaw thrust*, is usually more appropriate when resuscitation masks and devices are used or if a neck injury is suspected.

Jaw thrust

Head tilt and chin lift provide an open airway in most unconscious persons. However, if a neck injury is suspected, jaw thrust without head tilt is the safest initial approach to opening the airway since it can usually be accomplished without extending the neck. In addition, when an injured diver has a short, thick neck jaw thrust may be used.

Jaw thrust is achieved by applying pressure behind the angle of the jaw to gently thrust the jaw forward and open the mouth and airway. If a neck injury is suspected, the head should be carefully supported without tilting it backward or turning it from side to side. If jaw thrust alone is unsuccessful, the head should be tilted back slightly. Jaw thrust usually requires two hands.

FIGURE 3.2

Jaw thrust

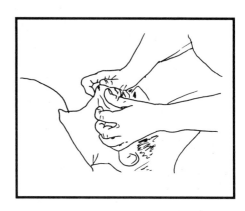

B - CHECK THE BREATHING

The next step is to determine whether or not the diver is breathing. This is done by *looking, listening and feeling for breathing.*

Lean down, place one ear near the injured diver's mouth and look towards the chest. From here you can look for movement of the lower chest and/or abdomen and, at the same time, listen and feel for breath coming out from the diver's mouth. Placing a hand lightly on the injured diver's chest or upper abdomen may make any breathing motions easier to detect. In addition, if a pair of glasses or some other clear glass or plastic object is held near the diver's mouth, it may fog up if the diver is exhaling, partly depending on environmental conditions.

Chest or abdomen movement alone only means that a person is trying to breathe. Such movement can occur for a limited time despite a blocked airway. It is important to feel for air coming out from the diver's mouth since this indicates movement of air to and from the lungs. Noisy breathing usually means there is some obstruction, since unobstructed breathing is normally relatively quiet.

To check for breathing:

- Look for the rise and fall of the chest and abdomen
- Feel for breath coming from the mouth
- Listen for breath coming from the mouth

Injured diver is breathing

If the injured diver is breathing adequately, place the diver in the recovery position with the head tilted backward and the mouth slightly downward. This position allows gravity to pull the tongue forward away from the back of the throat and opens the airway. It also allows drainage of fluid that has accumulated in the upper airways and reduces any obstruction by the palate and epiglottis. Supporting the chin will further open the airway. Positioning the thigh of the injured diver's top leg at right angles to the body, and bending the knee so that the calf is roughly parallel to the lower leg will help prevent the diver rolling forward onto the face.

FIGURE 3.3
Recovery position

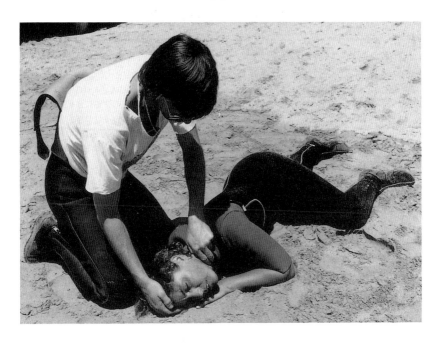

An unconscious, breathing diver should normally be placed in the recovery position (preferably on the left side if decompression illness is suspected), with the head tilted back and the chin supported. This will open up the airway and assist drainage of fluids, among other benefits.

C - CHECK THE CIRCULATION

Check the *carotid pulse* and note its rate and strength.

To check the carotid pulse:

- Place two or three fingers gently on the injured diver's Adam's Apple
- Slide these fingers into the groove on either side between the Adam's Apple and the large muscle of the neck
- Feel with the flat portion of the fingers (rather than the finger tips, which are less sensitive)
- Press gently inwards and backwards against the neck muscle

The carotid arteries, which supply blood to the brain, are large and close to the skin. The carotid pulse is taken since it is relatively easily detected when an injured person's blood vessels constrict with shock. Another relatively reliable pulse is the femoral pulse, located in the crease between the thigh and the abdomen. Pulses such as the radial (wrist) pulse become difficult to detect as blood vessels constrict with the onset of shock, or in response to cold environmental conditions.

It is important not to apply too much pressure on the carotid arteries because the blood supply to the brain may be impeded. In addition, excessive pressure on the carotid arteries may cause a reflex slowing of the heart and a subsequent drop in blood pressure (Carotid Sinus Syndrome). It is also important that only one carotid pulse is felt at a time.

The rate per minute can be determined by counting the number of beats in fifteen seconds and multiplying by four. Note whether the rhythm is regular or irregular and whether the beats are strong or feeble. Record the rate and strength since it will provide a reference with which to compare later readings and help determine whether or not the diver's condition is stable, improving or deteriorating. The normal resting pulse rate for an adult is between about 60 to 80 beats per minute. Athletes will generally have slower pulse rates. Pulse rates in an adult which remain above about 120 or below 50 may represent a serious problem. A rapid and weak pulse usually indicates that the person is in shock.

The injured diver should be shielded from the elements and insulated appropriately to maintain normal body temperature. *Supplemental oxygen should be provided as soon as possible.*

Diver is not breathing effectively

Inadequate respiration can be recognized by:

- the skin over the chest is sucked in causing the ribs to be exposed, and the abdomen rises (more common in children than adults and usually in cases of airway obstruction)
- rapid, shallow breathing, which may be noisy
- slow, shallow breathing, with bluish tinge to skin or mucous membranes

If the diver is making ineffective respiratory movements, recheck the airway, reapply head tilt/chin lift (or jaw thrust). If this fails to rectify the problem, commence rescue breathing. Weak respiratory movements will be easily overidden.

Absent respiration is recognized by:

- no apparent rise and fall of chest or abdomen
- cannot feel exhaled breath coming from mouth
- cannot hear breath coming from mouth
- diver may be cyanotic (i.e. the skin is a bluish color)

If the diver is not breathing effectively, rescue breathing should be commenced without delay and continued while any available oxygen equipment is being prepared for use.

RESCUE BREATHING (RB)

Mechanism of Rescue Breathing

TABLE 3.1

Composition of inspired and expired air		
	Inspired	Expired
Nitrogen	79%	79%
Oxygen	21%	16.5%
Carbon dioxide	0%	4%
Water vapor	0%	0.5%

As shown in Table 3.1, we use only a small proportion of the oxygen we inhale, so expired air still contains a substantial amount of oxygen. This oxygen concentration is sufficient to maintain consciousness and adequate oxygenation of the brain for a limited period.

RB involves a first aider using their expired breath to inflate the lungs and ventilate a non-breathing person. It is a very simple and highly effective method of providing an adequate supply of oxygen to a non-breathing person. The expired breath can be blown in through the injured person's mouth, nose, or both.

Mouth-to-mouth application is generally used by adults giving RB to other adults. In this case, the nose must be sealed. However, if mouth-to-mouth contact is ineffective (e.g. a seal cannot be obtained because loose dentures have been removed) or inappropriate (e.g. person swallowed poison or has mouth injuries) the mouth can be closed and RB applied via the injured person's nose.

It is often more hygenic and sometimes more effective to apply RB via an oronasal resuscitation mask or a face shield, as described in later chapters.

After ensuring a clear and open airway, seal the injured diver's nose with your fingers or cheek, inhale, seal your lips over the diver's mouth and gently blow your expired breath into the diver. *Blow just hard enough to cause the lower chest and abdomen to rise. Stop blowing as soon as the chest has risen and ensure that the chest is allowed to fall completely between each breath.* Initially, give two *slow* breaths, followed by 10 to 12 breaths per minute. Ventilations should take about one and a half to two seconds each.

During controlled ventilation, the first aider must ventilate strongly enough to ensure that the air or oxygen enters the injured diver's lungs, pushes down the diaphragm and expands the chest. To achieve this in an adult, a positive pressure of 15 to 20 cm of water (cmH_2O) is needed. This requires greater than normal tidal volumes. For example, the average adult, who has a tidal volume of around 500 ml, needs approximately 800 to 1200 ml to be adequately ventilated during controlled ventilation. Therefore, during rescue breathing a first aider must blow out approximately 60 to 240 percent more breath than they would normally exhale while at rest. Although this may appear to be a lot, it does not require much effort. The ventilations should normally be relatively gentle. However, if it is certain that the airway is maximally unobstructed and the injured diver's chest is still not rising sufficiently during inflations, stronger ventilations may be required. This may occur with the reduced lung compliance associated with near drowning and certain other disorders.

If the first aider ventilates too fast or too great a volume, their expired air may go down the esophagus and into the stomach (*gastric insufflation*) where it may cause *regurgitation*, which is discussed later in this chapter.

It is important to allow the chest to fall between inflations for two main reasons:

(1) If sufficient air is not allowed to escape before the next ventilation, pressure may build up in the upper airway, causing some air to go to the stomach.

(2) In a spontaneously breathing person, most gas exchange occurs on inhalation, when the capillaries are stretched and opened and the contact area between the alveoli and capillaries is maximized. However, during artificial ventilation (whether by RB, air bag or oxygen equipment) the reverse is true. During controlled ventilation, gas is forced into the alveoli with a positive pressure, expanding the alveoli, but at the same time compressing the pulmonary capillaries and reducing the blood flow through them. Therefore, during controlled ventilation, gas exchange during inspiration is less than during expiration when the pressure is relieved. Although some first aiders may believe that by vigorous positive pressure ventilation a greater volume of oxygen is forced into the injured person's bloodstream, in reality, the reverse may be true. This is another reason why it is important to allow the chest to fall completely before initiating the next breath.

METHOD OF RESCUE BREATHING

Position the injured diver on the back and open the airway by tilting the head right back and lifting the chin, or by jaw thrust.

If ventilating through the diver's mouth, seal their nose by pinching it closed with your fingers or sealing it with your cheek. Different techniques will be necessary on different injured persons.

Initially, blow in two slow ventilations of 1.5 to 2 seconds each, ensuring that the injured diver's chest rises and then falls completely between breaths. These initial breaths will partially reinflate collapsed alveoli, flush the lungs of some of the excess carbon dioxide and introduce a fresh supply of oxygen.

After these initial breaths, the first aider should check for the carotid pulse of the injured diver.

Normally, spend 5 to 10 seconds feeling for a pulse. However, if it is suspected that the diver is suffering from severe hypothermia, it is currently recommended to spend up to 30 to 45 seconds observing for respiration and pulse, since the effects of hypothermia cause the pulse and breathing to become very weak and slow and, therefore, difficult to detect.

FIGURE 3.4

Rescue breathing

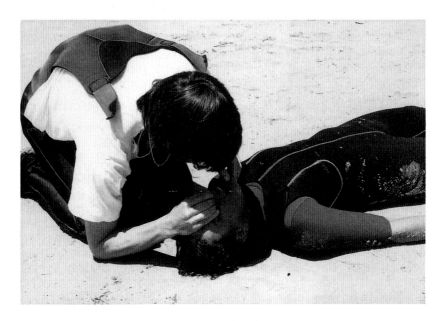

Pulse present

If you can feel a pulse but the diver is still breathless, continue to ventilate the diver at the rate of one breath every 5 to 6 seconds (10 to 12 ventilations per minute) for an adult, ensuring that the chest rises and then falls completely between ventilations. Do not overventilate the injured diver. As well as increasing the likelihood of gastric distension and regurgitation, it will cause you to hyperventilate and feel dizzy. If no pulse is apparent, CPR must be commenced (as described later).

Recheck the pulse (3 to 5 seconds) after about one minute and every few minutes thereafter. Ventilate the diver just before checking the pulse since the oxygen provided may cause the pulse to be stronger and more easily detected.

> **To perform RB:**
>
> - Activate the EMS
> - Place the injured diver flat on the back
> - Tilt the diver's head back and lift the jaw
> - Seal the diver's nose
> - Blow in two slow ventilations of 1.5 to 2 seconds each, ensuring the chest falls completely between ventilations
> - Check the carotid pulse (usually 5 to 10 seconds)
> - Ventilate at the rate of one breath every 5 to 6 seconds
> - Recheck the pulse after one minute and every few minutes thereafter

COMPLICATIONS WITH RESCUE BREATHING

1. Airway obstruction

If the airway is obstructed there will be resistance to inflation and the chest will not rise despite correct head tilt and jaw support. The most common cause of airway obstruction during RB is insufficient head tilt. If resistance is felt, the first thing to check is that the head tilt and jaw support are maximized. If the airway is still obstructed, it may be due to blockage by a foreign body or laryngospasm.

Inability to ventilate an unconscious diver is most likely due to improper technique since, in a diving situation, blockage from a solid object is unlikely. Visible liquids and semiliquids should be wiped out with the index and middle fingers covered by a piece of cloth; solid material should be extracted with a hooked index finger. However, if foreign body obstruction is strongly suspected, a series of abdominal or chest compressions can cause dislodgement of the object. The Heimlich Maneuver (subdiaphragmatic abdominal thrusts) is one method for removing a foreign body from the airway of an unconscious (or conscious) person.

Heimlich Maneuver with an unconscious, injured adult

The injured diver should be placed in a supine position. Kneeling astride the diver's thighs, the first aider places the heel of one hand against the injured diver's abdomen, in the midline slightly above the navel and well below the tip of the xiphoid process. The second hand is placed directly over the first and the first aider then presses into the abdomen with a quick upward thrust. The first aider must be positioned correctly to avoid thrusting to the right or left.

Regurgitation may be precipitated and should be dealt with as described below. If applied incorrectly, abdominal thrust techniques may damage internal organs such as the liver, spleen or stomach. The Heimlich Maneuver may be dangerous to a pregnant woman (who most diving physicians recommend should not be diving) and should be avoided in this situation. It may not be effective in a markedly obese person.

Chest thrusts can be used when the first aider cannot apply the Heimlich Maneuver effectively to the unconscious, markedly obese person (or in the late stages of pregnancy). The first aider should place the injured diver on the back and kneel close to the side of the injured diver's body. The hand position for the application of chest thrusts is the same as that for external chest compressions, described later. Each thrust should be delivered slowly, distinctly, and with the intent of relieving the obstruction.

Finger Sweep

"This maneuver should be used only in the unconscious victim, never in a seizure victim. With the victim face up, the rescuer should open the victim's mouth by grasping both the tongue and lower jaw between the thumb and fingers and lifting the mandible (tongue-jaw lift). This action draws the tongue away from the back of the throat and away from a foreign body that may be lodged there. This alone may partially relieve the obstruction. The rescuer inserts the index finger of the other hand down along the inside of the cheek and deeply into the throat to the base of the tongue. Then a hooking action is used to dislodge the foreign body and maneuver it into the mouth so that it can be removed. It is sometimes necessary to use the index finger to push the foreign body against the opposite side of the throat to dislodge and remove it. If the foreign body comes within reach, the rescuer should grasp and remove it. The rescuer must take care not to force the object deeper into the airway." (JAMA, 1992)

If a first aider is unable to ventilate an unconscious diver due to airway obstruction:

- Ensure maximum head tilt/chin lift and try to ventilate again
  If this is unsuccessful:
- Perform subdiaphragmatic abdominal thrusts (up to 5 times)
- Perform a finger sweep and attempt to ventilate again
  If this is unsuccessful:
- Repeat the sequence: thrusts, finger sweep and attempts to ventilate

---

Laryngospasm may completely or partially close the airway. It will eventually abate in adults, usually before irreparable brain damage occurs. If it is only partial, continue to blow air into the lungs to provide some oxygenation. Eventually, you may feel the resistance disappear as the spasm abates.

2. Regurgitation of stomach contents

An unconscious, non-breathing diver is usually placed in a supine position. In this position, the tongue can fall back and block the trachea. If the airway is not opened adequately and the diver is ventilated, the air will follow the path of least resistance. Since it is unable to enter the lungs, it will enter the esophagus. Overinflation of the lungs can also cause air to enter the esophagus.

At the level of the diaphragm there is a sphincter, known as the *cardiac sphincter*, which separates the esophagus and the stomach. In an adult, pressures greater than about 20 cmH_2O (which is a fairly low pressure) will cause this sphincter to open and force gas into the stomach. If too much pressure is generated in the airways and esophagus, gas will be forced into the stomach. This is known as *gastric insufflation*.

As gas enters the stomach, the stomach becomes distended and the pressure inside increases. If the pressure continues to increase, the cardiac sphincter will eventually open and allow the acidic gastric contents to flow up the esophagus and into the pharynx. This passive outflow of the stomach contents is called *regurgitation*, and, unfortunately, it is sometimes unavoidable. The gag reflex, which normally prevents foreign matter from entering the lungs, may not work at all in an unconscious diver and the acidic stomach contents may be allowed to enter the lungs. If the gastric contents are aspirated into the lungs, its acidity causes a very severe reaction which involves severe wheezing and cyanosis and complicates recovery.

Regurgitation is the passive outflow of stomach contents, often caused by gas entering the stomach during positive pressure ventilation.

Unlike vomiting, regurgitation is not accompanied by muscular spasm and is therefore more difficult for the first aider to detect. Resistance may suddenly be felt when ventilating the injured diver, or a gurgling sound might be heard. The stomach contents may be smelled or may be seen flowing into and out from the mouth.

When someone vomits, stomach contents are forcefully ejected by muscle spasm, which requires reasonable muscle tone. For this reason, vomiting (as opposed to regurgitation) only occurs when there is some level of consciousness. Therefore, *vomiting may be a positive sign during resuscitation since it often means that the injured diver is about to recommence breathing. In both regurgitation and vomiting the diver must be quickly turned onto the side, the airway cleared and breathing checked.*

Regurgitation can be precipitated in a number of ways during RB:

(1) If the airway is not adequately cleared or opened, relatively high pressures can build up as gas is blown into the narrowed airways. These pressures may rise enough to force air into the stomach.

It is important to clear the airway of obstructions and open it as widely as possible by using head tilt and jaw support, as appropriate. The airway should remain open during both ventilation and expiration.

(2) If excess gas is blown into the lungs, or if the flow rate is too rapid, sufficiently high pressures can be generated to force air into the stomach. This can occur as a result of overzealous inflation or failing to allow the chest to fall between inflations.

Inflation should cease as soon as the lower chest and abdomen rise, and the chest must be allowed to fall before the next ventilation.

(3) The first aider must take care not to put pressure on the stomach at any time.

If the injured diver's stomach becomes distended during RB, do not press on it to try to expel the gas since you will only increase the likelihood of regurgitation. Instead, try to rectify the cause of air entering the stomach by ensuring that the airway is clear and opened sufficiently, checking that you are not overventilating and that the chest is falling between inflations.

If the injured diver regurgitates, they should immediately be rolled onto the side and the airway cleared. Reposition the diver for ventilations, open the airway as far as possible and recommence resuscitation, taking care not to overinflate the diver's lungs.

Stomach inflation and regurgitation are less likely when:

- the airway is clear and opened widely during both ventilation and expiration
- ventilations are just sufficient to cause lower chest and abdomen to rise
- the chest is allowed to fall between inflations
- no pressure is placed on the stomach

Pulse absent

If the injured diver is unconscious, not breathing and a carotid pulse cannot be detected, it is likely that the heart has stopped beating effectively. This is known as *cardiac arrest. Absent carotid pulse is the main sign of cardiac arrest.*

Some resuscitation instructors have suggested that a first aider should lift the injured person's eye lids and observe whether or not the pupils constrict when exposed to light. Constriction of the pupils indicates that the heart is still beating, or that cardiac arrest has only occurred relatively recently. Unfortunately, this sign is not always reliable since a variety of factors, such as certain drugs and medications, may prevent the pupils from constricting even though the heart is beating. For this reason, this check is generally not recommended.

If the injured diver is cyanotic (i.e. the skin is blue) and cold, you may be more confident in the diagnosis of cardiac arrest. However, this is not always reliable, especially if the diver is suffering from hypothermia.

A diver who:

- is unconscious
- is not breathing
- **has no palpable carotid pulse**

is assumed to have cardiac arrest. Cardiopulmonary resuscitation (CPR) must be commenced at once.

CARDIOPULMONARY RESUSCITATION (CPR)

When the heart stops beating, the circulation of blood ceases (circulatory arrest) and, unless adequate artificial circulation and oxygenation are provided very quickly, brain tissues will begin to die (usually within about 4 minutes).

The most common form of cardiac arrest is known as *ventricular fibrillation*. During ventricular fibrillation, the heart muscle fibres contract and relax in an uncoordinated and irregular manner. Because the quivering heart cannot generate an effective pumping action, no pulse can be felt. When ventricular fibrillation occurs, it is necessary to use an electrical defibrillator, which applies an electric shock across the heart to stop the uncoordinated contractions and restore normal heartbeat.

While waiting for a medical aid to arrive with a defibrillator, artificial circulation should be provided by applying *external chest compressions* (ECC). Some recent studies on life support indicate that *the main factor determining the chances of survival after cardiac arrest is how quickly the heart is defibrillated*. Data from the United States have indicated that the highest hospital discharge rate has been achieved in those patients for whom CPR was initiated within 4 minutes of the time of the arrest and who, in addition, were provided with advanced cardiac life support within 8 minutes of their arrest. This is why it is so essential to activate the EMS rapidly.

If the first aider is alone and no one responds to their calls for help, it has previously been recommended that CPR should be performed for about one minute and then help should be summoned. (JAMA, 1986) However, revised guidelines have recently been released. These guidelines recommend that the EMS system be activated immediately unresponsiveness is determined in an adult victim, even if it means leaving the victim to do so. The following justification is offered:

"A potential concern about activating the EMS system before full assessment (by the single trained rescuer) is the delay incurred in treating the patient with primary respiratory arrest or an obstructed airway. In many adult patients with primary respiratory compromise - such as asphyxiation, drowning, strangulation, respiratory arrest due to epileptic seizures, drug overdoses, or obstructed airway - airway opening and rescue breathing are indicated, not chest compression or defibrillation. However, even trained rescuers may be unable to distinguish between primary cardiac arrest and a collapse secondary to airway and breathing problems. In addition, the vast majority of sudden death victims will not have a primary obstructed airway. More than 80% of such victims of out-of-hospital cardiac arrest will be in ventricular fibrillation, and defibrillation is the key to survival in such patients. Hence for all adult patients, activating the EMS system immediately after determining unresponsiveness is justified." (JAMA, 1992)

In certain diving situations, where cardiac arrest is often only secondary to airway compromise (and neck injuries are rare), it may sometimes be appropriate for the lone first aider to quickly but carefully roll the injured diver into the recovery position before leaving to activate the EMS. This may offer some protection to the airway in the event the diver is breathing, begins to breathe and/or vomits.

It is important to make a careful effort to detect the carotid pulse prior to commencing ECC, since performing chest compressions on an injured diver who has a pulse may result in serious medical complications.

In the event of cardiac arrest:

- Activate the EMS without delay
- Do not leave the injured diver unless there is no choice
- Commence CPR as soon as possible

Remember: The main factor determining the chances of survival after cardiac arrest is how quickly the heart is defibrillated. However, defibrillation is more likely to be successful if effective CPR has been commenced soon after cardiac arrest.

MECHANISM OF EXTERNAL CHEST COMPRESSIONS

During external chest compressions, the first aider places their hands (one on top of the other for an adult injured person) over the lower half of the sternum (breastbone) and compresses the chest rhythmically.

Although there is some dispute about the exact mechanism of external cardiac compressions, it appears that intermittently pressing the sternum downward produces some blood flow by a combination of the following mechanisms:

(1) The heart may be squeezed between the sternum and the spine causing an increased pressure in the ventricles. If the valves between the atria and ventricles close, blood will be ejected into the pulmonary artery and aorta. This is particulary likely when the heart is relatively large and the chest is compliant, as in children.

(2) When the chest is compressed, the pressure is increased throughout the entire chest. A pressure gradient is established between various organs and vessels within the chest and those outside the chest. Blood is forced from the heart, lungs and major blood vessels due to the valves of the major veins at the inlet to the chest, and flows to the carotid arteries and various other vessels outside the chest. When the pressure is released and the chest expands, the pressure gradient is reversed and blood returns to the chest. In this situation, the heart acts as a conduit, directing the blood flow to various organs. This is more likely to occur when the chest is large and the pressure of compressions relatively light.

Positioning the injured diver

The injured diver requiring resuscitation must be placed supine on a firm, horizontal surface. If the surface is not firm, compressions will not be effective. Boards can be placed under the diver to provide firm support. The head must not be elevated above the heart or potential blood flow to the brain will be further reduced.

Locating the compression point

The recommended compression point is on the mid-line over the lower half of the sternum. The following guidelines may be used to identify the lower sternum:

"1. The rescuer's hand locates the lower margin of the victim's rib cage on the side next to the rescuer.

2. The fingers are then moved up the rib cage to the notch where the ribs meet the sternum in the center of the lower part of the chest.

3. The heel of one hand is placed on the lower half of the sternum and the other hand is placed on top of the hand on the sternum so that the hands are parallel. The long axis of the heel of the rescuer's hand should be placed on the long axis

of the sternum. This will keep the main force of compression on the sternum and decrease the chance of rib fracture.

4. The fingers may be either extended or interlaced but must be kept off the chest.

5. Because of the varying sizes and shapes of different person's hands, an alternate acceptable hand position is to grasp the wrist of the hand on the chest with the hand that has been locating the lower end of the sternum. This technique is helpful for rescuers with arthritic problems of the hands and wrists." (JAMA, 1992)

To locate the compression point:

- Find the lower end of the sternum by following the bottom rib to the notch where it meets the sternum.
- Place the heel of one hand on the lower half of the sternum so that the long axis of the heel of your hand is on the long axis of the sternum. Place the other hand on top of the first so that the hands are parallel.
- The hands should be about one finger's width above the bottom of the sternum.

It is important to ensure that the hands are not positioned too low when performing ECC to avoid injuries to underlying organs. Attached to the bottom of the sternum is a structure known as the *xiphoid process*. The xiphoid is made of cartilage and is easily dislocated and possibly broken if pressure is exerted on it. A displaced xiphoid could rupture underlying organs. In addition, if the hands are too low, pressure may be applied to the stomach and regurgitation may result.

Ribs are easily broken during ECC if too much pressure is exerted on them. A broken rib can puncture a lung or damage other underlying organs. *To minimize the likelihood of breaking ribs, ensure that you keep your fingers off the chest and only apply pressure on the sternum with the heel of the palm of your hand.* Ensure that pressure is applied vertically over the sternum by positioning yourself right beside the injured diver's chest and positioning your shoulders directly above the compression point. If the thrust is not in a straight downward direction, the torso has a tendency to roll, part of the force is lost and the compressions may be less effective. In addition, try to make the compressions smooth rather than jerky. Keeping the elbows stiff helps to achieve smoother compressions and reduce first aider fatigue.

Although the pressure on the chest should be completely released between compressions, the hands should not be lifted from the chest. Leaving the hands lightly on the chest between compressions enables smoother compressions.

Ribs may be broken without the first aider realizing, and sometimes it is impossible to avoid breaking ribs, especially in the elderly. However, effective circulation with broken ribs is better than intact ribs and inadequate circulation. Other complications may occur despite proper CPR technique. These include fracture of the sternum, separation of the ribs from the sternum, pneumothorax, lacerations of the liver and spleen, and others. These complications may be minimized by careful attention to details of performance, but they cannot entirely be prevented. Accordingly, concern for injuries that may result from properly performed CPR should not impede the prompt and energetic application of CPR.

When performing external chest compressions:

- Ensure the compressions are smooth and rythmical
- Ensure the pressure is applied directly over the sternum and not to the ribs

---

FIGURE 3.5

Hand position for external chest compression

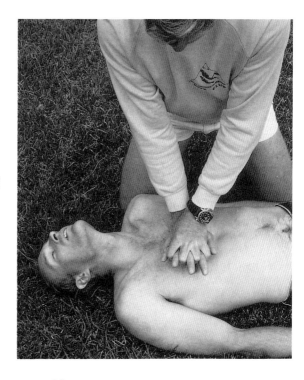

Depth of compression

The depth of sternal compression on an adult is around 1.5 to 2 inches. The first few compressions can be a bit lighter to gauge the spring and strength of the sternum.

If possible, get someone to feel for the injured diver's artificially generated carotid pulse soon after you begin performing ECC so you know that you are generating circulation. If no artificial pulse is detected, the compressions may not be forceful enough, the compressor's hand position may be incorrect, or the other first aider may not have found the carotid artery. Optimal sternal compression is best gauged by using the compression force that generates a palpable carotid or femoral pulse.

Compression/release ratio

The chest must be allowed to recoil between compressions to allow blood to return to the heart and other vessels in the chest. Some evidence indicates that arterial pressure during chest compression is maximal when the duration of compression is 50% of the compression-release cycle. A first aider should aim to achieve a compression-release cycle of 50:50 when performing ECC.

Rate of compression

Over the years, there has been some debate about the optimum rate of chest compression.

The previously recommended 60 compressions per minute originally arose from what seemed reasonable for a living person. However, because of the physiological changes that are underway in the person being resuscitated, CPR rates derived from normal pulse rates may not be optimal.

Certain studies indicated that rates slower than 60 beats per minute did not reduce the blood flow in the carotid and femoral arteries as long as the compressions were sustained for 60% of the compression-release cycle. Other studies have shown that increasing the compression rate can lead to an increase in blood flow in the carotid arteries. In addition, it has been demonstrated that increasing the rate above 60 cycles per minute can increase the blood flow to the coronary arteries themselves.

Currently, a rate of 80 to 100 compressions per minute is recommended for an adult injured person.

External chest compressions are combined with positive pressure ventilations to perform *cardiopulmonary resuscitation* (CPR).

CPR is applied to an injured person who has had a cardiac arrest (i.e. unconscious, not breathing and has no pulse). It can be performed by a single person or by multiple rescuers.

SINGLE RESCUER CPR

When CPR is performed by a single rescuer on an adult, the rescuer must perform cycles of two ventilations followed by 15 compressions, with a compression rate of 80-100 per minute.

The ventilations should be applied relatively slowly (1.5 to 2 seconds each), *ensuring that the chest falls between ventilations.*

CPR is stopped to recheck the carotid pulse for 3 to 5 seconds after the first four cycles. If a pulse is still absent, CPR is resumed. If CPR is continued, it should be stopped to check for a returned pulse and spontaneous breathing every few minutes. CPR should not be interrupted except in special circumstances. Although it is unlikely that a spontaneous pulse will have returned, it may occasionally do so, especially in situations such as a witnessed near drowning where the diver was rapidly recovered and resuscitation was commenced immediately.

If a pulse is detected, the breathing is then checked (usually 3 to 5 seconds). If there is a pulse but no breathing, rescue breathing should be commenced at a rate of 10 to 12 breaths per minute and the pulse should be monitored carefully. However, if breathing is present, the diver should be placed in the recovery position (if no neck injury is suspected or evident), and the airway, breathing and pulse should be monitored carefully.

If CPR is applied effectively, the injured diver may become less cyanotic and the skin color may become more normal.

TWO RESCUER CPR

When two rescuers trained in CPR are available, both can be involved in the resuscitation. This is potentially much more effective. One rescuer manages the airway and ventilates the injured diver, while the other compresses the chest. The rescuers can change roles periodically to prevent excessive fatigue.

With two rescuer CPR, one ventilation (of 1.5 to 2 seconds) should be given after every 5 compressions. There should be a pause in the compressions to allow the ventilation. Exhalation occurs during compressions. The compression rate is 80-100 per minute.

If the compressor counts up to five aloud, the person ventilating will know when to interpose the breath. Counting in thousands helps to time the seconds. i.e. One thousand, two thousand, three thousand, four thousand, five thousand - *stop for breath* - one thousand ....

The rescuers must ensure that the chest is not being compressed when the ventilation is given. Certain experiments have indicated that better cerebral circulation may be achieved when the injured person is ventilated at the same time as a compression is given. However, this practice has also been shown to reduce blood flow to the coronary arteries. In addition, simultaneous ventilations will increase the likelihood of gastric distension, thereby causing regurgitation with all its associated complications. *Therefore, compressing and ventilating the diver simultaneously should be avoided. It is avoided by interrupting the compressions when the ventilation is given.*

The ratios, rate and depth for CPR on an adult diver are:

- **1 rescuer** - 2 breaths and 15 compressions
- **2 rescuers** - 1 breath and 5 compressions

- Rate of compression - 80 to 100 per minute
- Depth of compression - 1.5 to 2 inches

CPR performed by two rescuers can be far more effective than single rescuer CPR since a more continuous circulation can be achieved and rescuer exhaustion is less likely.

Some studies have indicated that, even when performed correctly, standard CPR results in a cardiac output, carotid artery blood flow and cerebral blood flow usually less than 30% of normal. Since this is just sufficient to prevent brain damage there is no margin for inefficient methods. This is why it is so beneficial to supplement CPR with the provision of high concentrations of oxygen.

The effectiveness of the compressions can be checked by feeling for the artificially generated carotid pulse while compressions are being done. This is done by the person who is managing the airway and ventilating the injured diver. The artificial pulse should be checked soon after compressions have begun to ensure that the compressions are deep enough. If no generated pulse is detected, the compressions may not be forceful enough, the compressor's hand position may be incorrect or the person feeling for the pulse may not have found the carotid artery.

Improvement in the diver's lip and face color indicates that both the ventilations and compressions are effective. However, you should not be discouraged by a lack of improvement in color. Check your technique and continue CPR until medical assistance arrives.

As previously mentioned, CPR is stopped to recheck the carotid pulse for 3 to 5 seconds after the first four cycles and thereafter every few minutes. Just before the compressions are stopped for the periodic pulse check, the rescuer managing the airway can locate the artificially generated carotid pulse and leave their fingers there. The other rescuer then stops the compressions while the first rescuer continues to feel for a pulse for 5 seconds. If a spontaneous pulse is now felt, ventilations are maintained and the pulse is monitored, but ECC is discontinued. If no pulse is felt, CPR is recommenced.

A first aider should continue CPR until one of the following occurs: "(1) effective spontaneous circulation and ventilation have been restored; (2) care is transferred to emergency medical responders or another trained person who continues basic life support; (3) care is transferred to advanced life support emergency medical personnel; (4) care is transferred to a physician who determines that resuscitation should be discontinued; (5) reliable criteria for the determination of death are recognized; (6) the rescuer is too exhausted to continue resuscitation, environmental hazards endanger the rescuer, or continued resuscitation would jeopardize the lives of others; (7) a valid no-CPR order is presented to the rescuers." (JAMA, 1992)

The effectiveness of CPR can be monitored by:

- improvement in the color of the diver
- presence of an artificial pulse (2 rescuers)
- return of a spontaneous pulse

Note:

It is not appropriate to perform external chest compressions without ventilations.

REVIEW QUESTIONS

1. Why is it important to commence resuscitation as soon as possible, when required?

2. Why is it important to handle an unconscious diver gently?

3. What is the preferred method to open the airway?

4. Why is it important to support the chin of an unconscious diver?

5. Why is an unconscious, breathing diver positioned on the side?

6. List the information to be relayed to the EMS in a resuscitation emergency.

7. How hard should a first aider ventilate when performing rescue breathing?

8. Why is it important to allow the chest to fall between ventilations?
9. With an unconscious diver, which pulse is checked and for how long?
10. What is the recommended method to clear an obstruction from the airway?
11. What can cause air to enter a diver's stomach during resuscitation?
12. How can a first aider distinguish between regurgitation and vomiting?
13. What action is taken if a diver regurgitates?
14. What is the main sign of cardiac arrest?
15. What are the ratios and rates for single-rescuer CPR on an adult?
16. What are the ratios and rates for two-rescuer CPR on an adult?
17. How can the effectiveness of RB be monitored?
18. How can the effectiveness of CPR be monitored?

CPR SEQUENCE

1. Check environment for hazards (to first aider and injured diver)
2. Determine level of consciousness:
   - speak to injured diver
   - gently shake diver
3. Activate the EMS immediately
4. Head tilt/chin lift or jaw thrust, as appropriate
5. Check for signs of respiratory failure:
   - look for chest/abdomen rise and fall
   - feel for injured diver's breath
   - listen for diver's breath
6. If diver is breathing, place in recovery position and monitor ABC
7. If diver is not breathing effectively, seal the nose, and then:
8. Give two full ventilations of 1.5 to 2 seconds each
9. Check carotid pulse
10. If pulse present, continue ventilations (one every 5 to 6 seconds) and monitor pulse
11. If pulse absent, locate correct compression point (center of lower sternum)
12. Commence CPR:
    one rescuer   - 15 compressions/2 breaths
    two rescuers - 5 compressions/1 breath

    Compression rate 80 to 100 per minute
    Depth of compressions 1.5 to 2 inches for adult
13. Recheck carotid pulse after first four cycles and then every few minutes
14. If diver regurgitates, roll onto side, clear mouth, reposition on back, tilt head, lift jaw, ventilate gently ensuring chest rises and then falls completely before giving the next breath
15. If diver vomits, roll onto side, clear mouth and check for breathing
16. Following revival, place diver in recovery position and treat for shock
17. Confirm that EMS has been activated.

Chapter 4

BENEFITS OF BREATHING ELEVATED OXYGEN CONCENTRATIONS

The amount of oxygen delivered to a tissue depends on the quantity of oxygen in the blood and the rate of blood flow (perfusion). Since the hemoglobin is normally almost fully saturated, the blood usually cannot carry much more oxygen bonded to hemoglobin. However, in certain disorders, the performance of the lungs in delivering oxygen to the blood is impaired, leading to a reduction in hemoglobin saturation. In these circumstances, increasing the inspired oxygen concentration can significantly increase the hemoglobin saturation. In addition, when an elevated concentration of oxygen is breathed, the higher partial pressure of oxygen causes more of it to dissolve into the plasma of the blood (in accordance with Henry's Law). By maximizing the inspired oxygen concentration we can maximize the hemoglobin saturation and increase the amount of oxygen dissolved in plasma. This increases the chances of survival of tissues with a poor blood supply, as well as other weakened tissues. Consequently, additional oxygen is important in the management of shock and resuscitation. Oxygen is the agent of choice in the first aid and treatment of many types of diving-related injuries, especially decompression illness.

THE BENEFITS OF HIGH OXYGEN CONCENTRATIONS IN THE FIRST AID FOR DIVING ACCIDENTS

As mentioned previously, the breathing of high concentrations of oxygen plays an important role in the management of diving accidents. The reasons for this will be briefly outlined in the following section.

Decompression illness

Decompression illness (DCI) is a new classification used to describe decompression sickness and cerebral arterial gas embolism. Because the manifestations and the treatment of the two disorders are often identical, and because of the difficulty of distinguishing between them, some diving physicians have now classified them as one.

Decompression illness results from the formation of gas bubbles (usually nitrogen or air) in the blood and body tissues. These bubbles can distort and disrupt tissues, block or damage blood vessels and cause biochemical changes in the blood. The location and volume of the bubbles determines the type of symptoms and the severity of the illness.

Signs and symptoms of DCI include: extreme fatigue, numbness, tingling, headache, pain in joints, other body pain, weakness, vision or speech difficulty, decreased consciousness, incoordination, paralysis and many others.

Breathing 100% oxygen provides very important benefits for a diver suffering from DCI. These are:

- By eliminating nitrogen from the inspired gas, 100% oxygen breathing speeds up nitrogen elimination from the body, thus reducing bubble size more quickly.

    A gas diffuses from an area of high concentration to areas of lower concentration. The greater the difference in concentrations of the gas, the faster this diffusion occurs. When breathing 100% oxygen, the injured diver is not inhaling the large amounts of nitrogen present in air. Washing out nitrogen from the lungs encourages the nitrogen in the blood to diffuse into the lungs and lowers the partial pressure of nitrogen in the arterial blood. This arterial blood then passes through the tissues, and, since it now contains much less nitrogen than the tissues, nitrogen diffuses from the tissues and from the bubbles into the blood and is taken to the lungs and eliminated. This cycle continues until all the excess nitrogen is removed. The effect is reduced greatly as the inspired oxygen level falls below 100%.

- Any reduction in blood flow due to bubble formation may cause hypoxia in affected tissues. The higher oxygen partial pressures will help to oxygenate any hypoxic tissues.

- Higher oxygen concentrations can help compensate for hypoxemia resulting from impaired gas transfer from the lungs to the blood and reduce any hypoxic respiratory distress.

- Higher oxygen concentrations may help reduce the shock and cerebral edema that may be associated with decompression illness.

    Recent research indicates that hyperbaric oxygen may inhibit the accumulation of white blood cells in areas where there is a deficiency of blood flow. These cells will both block blood vessels and cause tissue damage via toxic chemicals that they produce.

Pulmonary barotrauma (ruptured lung)

If the expanding air in a diver's lungs cannot escape quickly enough during ascent, areas of lung may overdistend and tear. Air will escape from the damaged lung(s) and enter various body cavities and tissues. The diver will suffer from hypoxemia as a result of the reduced efficiency of the lungs. In addition, the escaping air may cause problems, depending on where it collects. If it collects in the mediastinum (mediastinal emphysema), it can cause chest pain and occasionally can affect heart action. If it collects in the loose tissue of the neck (subcutaneous emphysema) it can affect speech and can cause difficulty swallowing or breathing. If it escapes into the pleural cavity, the two layers of pleura will no longer be in contact and the lung may pull away from the chest wall and collapse (pneumothorax). Rupture into a blood vessel results in arterial gas (air) embolism.

Symptoms of pulmonary barotrauma include: chest pain, shortness of breath, coughing, cyanosis, shock, voice changes and difficulty swallowing.

Breathing 100% oxygen can reduce the hypoxemia associated with pulmonary barotrauma by increasing the transfer of oxygen across damaged or poorly perfused lung surface, thereby offsetting the impairment due to the damage. In addition, by nitrogen elimination, oxygen breathing reduces the volume of escaped air trapped in the chest cavity and leads to a more rapid resolution of symptoms.

FIGURE 4.1
An injured diver receiving oxygen

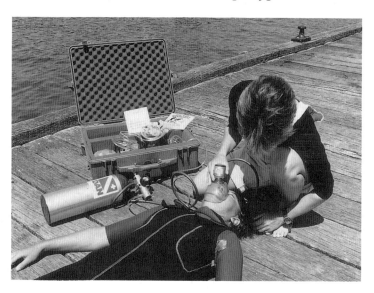

Carbon monoxide toxicity

Carbon monoxide, which may be a contaminant in a diver's breathing air, exerts major toxic effects on the brain. In addition to these toxic effects, a victim of carbon monoxide poisoning may suffer the effects of hypoxia.

Carbon monoxide combines far more readily with hemoglobin than oxygen does. This reduces the major means of oxygen transport through the body and may lead to hypoxia.

Signs and symptoms of carbon monoxide toxicity include: headache, dizziness, nausea, vomiting, confusion, memory loss, breathlessness, weakness, incoordination, loss of balance, unconsciousness and death.

Increasing the concentration of inspired oxygen helps to break the bond between the carbon monoxide and hemoglobin and other tissue proteins. In addition, oxygen breathing enables more oxygen to dissolve into the blood plasma, thereby improving the oxygen supply to the tissues.

Near drowning and salt water aspiration syndrome

Water entering the throat normally causes a reflex spasm of the larynx to prevent water entering the lungs. However, factors such as alcohol, certain drugs and unconsciousness can inhibit this reflex. Hypoxia will eventually cause the spasm to abate in adults. In simple terms, if the spasm abates while the person is still submerged, water will enter the trachea, pass into the lungs and displace lung air with water. Gas exchange will cease, leading to severe hypoxemia and subsequent tissue hypoxia.

Large quantities of water are not required to disrupt lung function. Death may occur during the primary incident, or later as a result of the adverse effects of water inhalation on lung surfactant and alveolar lining cells (secondary drowning), from cerebral hypoxia and/or shock, secondary to prolonged hypoxia, or to pneumonia, resulting from the inhalation of foreign matter. Many victims will have a stomach full of water and resuscitation can often be complicated by the regurgitation of stomach contents. A person who survives is generally said to have near drowned. One who cannot be resuscitated has drowned.

Hypoxemia is the most important consequence of near drowning. The duration of hypoxia is the critical factor in determining the victim's outcome.

If a diver fails to clear the regulator or snorkel adequately, or if the regulator is leaking, a fine mist of salt water may be inhaled. The water can cause acute inflammation of the alveoli which produces the effects of salt water aspiration syndrome. Salt water aspiration syndrome is often considered a mild form of near drowning. The affected diver often suffers an immediate cough. Then, there is usually a latent period before further manifestations occur. Delayed signs and symptoms include: shortness of breath, coughing, chest pain, uncontrollable shivering, fever and mild hypoxia.

As mentioned, conditions such as near drowning and salt water aspiration reduce the oxygen uptake from the lungs and cause various degrees of respiratory distress, leading to tissue hypoxia. Breathing elevated concentrations of oxygen helps to reduce the symptoms of hypoxia.

Hypothermia

When a diver suffers from hypothermia, circulation is reduced to the peripheral tissues to reduce heat loss. If heat loss continues, eventually the heart slows down and the blood thickens. Although vital organs are protected to some extent, hypoxia of the brain develops.

Signs and symptoms of hypothermia include: numbness, blotchy or blue skin, shivering, depressed mental function, incoordination, muscle stiffness, cessation of shivering, absent reflexes, depressed breathing and pulse, heart irregularities and death.

"It is important to prevent further heat loss from the patient's body core by removing wet garments from the victim, insulating the victim, shielding him or her from wind, and ventilating with warm, humidified oxygen." (JAMA, 1992)

Provision of higher concentrations of externally warmed, humidified oxygen has been used effectively to treat hypothermia. Currently, there is uncertainty as to whether breathing warmed oxygen actually helps to reheat the core, or whether it simply reduces the heat loss from respiration. However, the additional oxygen will help offset the hypoxia resulting from hypothermia.

Special equipment must be used to deliver warmed, humidified oxygen since the oxygen delivered by normal delivery systems will be relatively cool and dry.

Marine animal envenomation

Envenomation by marine animals such as the stingray, stonefish, jellyfish, sea snake and blue ringed octopus (found in the Indo-Pacific region) can cause varying degrees of respiratory depression. Provision of high concentrations of inspired oxygen helps to offset the resulting hypoxia.

Shock

Shock occurs when the circulation is inadequate to meet the oxygen demands of the major body organs. It accompanies many injuries. The resulting hypoxia can be partly offset by increasing the concentration of the inspired oxygen, since more oxygen will be carried by the blood.

Resuscitation

Some studies have indicated that, even when performed correctly, standard CPR results in a cardiac output, carotid artery blood flow and cerebral blood flow usually less than 30% of normal. Since this is just sufficient to prevent brain damage there is no margin for inefficient methods. By raising the blood oxygen levels, oxygen-supplemented rescuscitation will help offset the reduced ventilation and perfusion that occur prior to, and during, resuscitation.

In summary, 100% oxygen provides the following benefits to the diver:

- adds no more inert gas
- washes out dissolved nitrogen
- washes out the nitrogen in bubbles, thus reducing bubble size
- improves blood and tissue oxygenation
- helps reduce respiratory distress
- may reduce shock and cerebral edema

FIGURE 4.2
Oxygen resuscitation

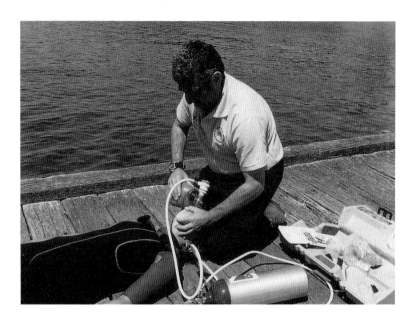

The benefits of providing higher inspired concentrations of oxygen to injured divers are substantial. However, using equipment in providing first aid introduces new potential problems and responsibilities, many of which are outlined throughout this book.

REVIEW QUESTIONS

1. List six of the more common manifestations of decompression illness.

2. List the benefits of breathing high oxygen concentrations for a diver suffering from decompression illness.

3. List four of the more general manifestations of pulmonary barotrauma.

4. List the benefits of breathing high oxygen concentrations for a diver suffering from pulmonary barotrauma.

5. What are the benefits of breathing high oxygen concentrations for a diver suffering from carbon monoxide toxicity.

Chapter 5

WHEN TO PROVIDE OXYGEN TO A DIVER

Most divers requiring oxygen provision will be breathing and, usually, conscious. It is important to reassure the injured diver and explain what you are doing. In the United States, an oxygen provider must obtain permission from the injured diver before providing oxygen. Permission can be sought by saying something to the effect of: *"This is oxygen. It will make you feel better. May I help you?"*. For unconscious divers, permission is assumed.

If decompression illness is suspected, the injured diver should be positioned horizontally without the head or legs elevated. If the diver feels faint, has a thready pulse or low blood pressure, elevation of the legs may raise the blood pressure. However, if the injured diver's condition appears to deteriorate as a result, the legs should be lowered.

Unconscious or nauseated divers should be placed on the side to prevent aspiration of vomitus and facilitate an open airway. Any diver requiring resuscitation should be placed supine and resuscitation procedures should be commenced immediately while the oxygen equipment is being prepared.

Some injured divers, such as those suffering from a heart attack, may find it difficult to breathe while lying flat and may find it easier to breathe while sitting or semi-reclined.

Oxygen breathing should be commenced as soon as possible after an accident to gain the maximum benefit. **If only a limited supply of oxygen is available, it should be given in maximum inspired concentrations from the time the accident is recognized until the supply of oxygen is exhausted.**

Oxygen provision should normally only be interrupted temporarily if the diver vomits, regurgitates, during a seizure or when the supply is depleted. Oxygen provision should be resumed at the earliest possible moment.

Ideally, all divers should have access to oxygen should it be needed after a dive. The sooner an injured diver receives oxygen, the better.

Divers Alert Network (DAN) data from the United States indicate that many divers are not receiving adequate oxygen first aid in the field. Oxygen as a first aid measure was provided in only 31 to 37 percent of the diving accident cases reported to DAN (USA) from 1987 to 1991.

All dive charter boats, dive training facilities and other commercial diving operations should carry oxygen equipment capable of delivering 100% oxygen to a breathing or non-breathing diver and ensure that their staff are adequately trained and qualified to use it.

In the Final Summary of Recommendations from the 1990 Undersea and Hyperbaric Medical Society Diving Accident Workshop it is stated:

"... It is further suggested that dive instructors and dive masters who are responsible for conducting dives be trained in the use of oxygen. The absence of an individual trained in oxygen administration should not preclude equipping a given dive boat with oxygen apparatus..."

Oxygen breathing should not be considered a final treatment for diving emergencies. It is part of normal diving first aid procedures and should increase the effectiveness of those procedures, giving the diver the greatest chance of a full and speedy recovery. Even though a diver may appear to have improved greatly or even completely since breathing oxygen, the diver must still receive immediate diving medical specialist attention. Although the immediate symptoms may have disappeared, the underlying cause may still be present.

The breathing of oxygen is only a first aid measure and is not a substitute for full medical evaluation and treatment for any diving injury. It must never be substituted for the recompression required for decompression illness, regardless of the diver's response.

REVIEW QUESTIONS

1. How should a diver suffering from decompression illness be positioned?
2. How soon after a diving accident should oxygen provision commence?
3. For how long should oxygen be provided?
4. When is oxygen provision interrupted?
5. Why should a diver be recompressed, even if symptoms of decompression illness may have disappeared during oxygen first aid?

Chapter 6

ADVERSE REACTIONS TO OXYGEN

OXYGEN TOXICITY

Oxygen breathed at partial pressures greater than about 0.6 ATA may become toxic under certain circumstances. Toxicity mainly depends on the partial pressure of oxygen and the length of exposure.

PULMONARY OXYGEN TOXICITY

Continual breathing of 100% oxygen at the surface may cause irritation of the respiratory tract and lungs within 24 hours. This is known as *pulmonary oxygen toxicity*. Symptoms such as pain behind the breastbone followed by coughing, wheezing and shortness of breath may occur. However, lower concentrations can be breathed for longer periods before causing ill-effects.

Pulmonary oxygen toxicity does not normally present a problem for the recreational diver unless recompression for decompression illness is required. During recompression, the diver will breathe very high oxygen concentrations for a number of hours. If, prior to recompression, there had been a very long delay (longer than about 5 hours) during which the diver breathed 100% oxygen continuously, pulmonary oxygen toxicity could become a consideration. The treating hyperbaric physician will consider this when deciding treatment options.

The risk of pulmonary oxygen toxicity can be reduced by ensuring the diver breathes air for 5 minutes after every 25 minutes on 100% oxygen. These air breaks minimize the toxic effect that elevated oxygen concentrations have on the lungs.

Most facilities are not concerned about air breaks during pre-hospital transport since the injured diver usually does not breathe 100% oxygen for such prolonged periods. In addition, the inspired oxygen concentration is unfortunately often far lower than 100% due to the type of delivery system used or a poor mask seal.

Periods of oxygen breathing should be recorded and the diver's response to oxygen should also be recorded and relayed to the treating hyperbaric physician.

CENTRAL NERVOUS SYSTEM (CNS) OXYGEN TOXICITY

When oxygen is breathed at partial pressures usually (but not always) greater than about 1.6 ATA it produces toxicity relatively rapidly and affects the brain, sometimes causing epileptic-like convulsions. This is known as *central nervous system (CNS)* or *acute neurological oxygen toxicity*. A diver breathing air would have to go to a depth of 218 feet (66 metres) in order to reach an oxygen partial pressure of 1.6 ATA. The likelihood of CNS oxygen toxicity increases with oxygen partial pressure, exposure time, exercise, cold, anxiety and increasing carbon dioxide levels in the blood. Animal studies suggest that nitrogen may enhance the onset of CNS oxygen toxicity, but the precise effects in man are not yet clear.

Some commercial, scientific, cave and deep wreck divers breathe pure oxygen in the water while decompressing. They do so to either reduce their decompression time or to add a safety margin to their air decompression calculations. If these divers were to descend beyond about 20 feet (6 metres) while breathing oxygen, they would risk acute oxygen toxicity. However, as previously mentioned, the depth of onset varies greatly between individuals and depends on other factors such as exertion, cold and time of exposure. Some naval divers routinely decompress breathing pure oxygen at 30 feet (9 metres), but they often wear a full-face mask. A diver, not wearing a full-face mask, who convulses underwater, would probably drown.

Some military, scientific and the so-called "technical" divers use mixtures of breathing gas (enriched air nitrox, heliox or trimix) which contain a higher percentage of oxygen than is in air. To avoid CNS oxygen toxicity, these divers must test the breathing mixture and very carefully calculate equivalent air depths, maximum allowable partial pressures of oxygen and exposure times to high partial pressures of oxygen as part of their comprehensive pre-dive preparation. Special tables of oxygen exposure limits are available.

A recreational diver would normally not be exposed to the risk of CNS oxygen toxicity unless being treated for decompression illness or possibly carbon monoxide toxicity. Routine treatment for decompression illness involves breathing 100% oxygen at a partial pressure of 2.8 ATA, which is equivalent to being at a depth of 60 feet of sea water (fsw) on pure oxygen. During recompression, the diver is carefully monitored for signs of toxicity and the oxygen level is reduced if necessary. In addition, convulsions are far less likely to occur at rest and in a dry chamber rather than in the water.

Hyperventilation

Some people hyperventilate (overbreathe) when they become anxious and such people may have difficulty breathing oxygen from a demand system while hyperventilating. The injured diver's rapid demands for breath may not easily be met due to the breathing resistance of the demand valve. This may increase the anxiety and magnify the problem. Consequently, if any rapidly breathing diver has difficulty breathing from a demand valve, the oxygen provider should reassure the diver and wait until their breathing slows sufficiently before trying the demand valve again. In the meantime, oxygen can be provided using a constant flow system. The diver's rapid breathing rate will reduce the inspired oxygen concentration delivered with certain constant flow delivery devices (e.g. those without a reservoir bag).

Transient worsening of symptoms

Occasionally, the symptoms of a diver suffering from decompression illness may worsen transiently shortly after oxygen is provided. Although the cause of this is still unclear, several possible explanations have been offered. These include: (1) oxygen rapidly diffusing into and temporarily increasing the size of existing bubbles before substantial nitrogen has diffused from the bubble; (2) shrinking bubbles relocating to an area where they cause further symptoms; and/or (3) oxygen breathing may cause peripheral blood vessels to constrict, thereby reducing the blood flow to affected areas and possibly causing some symptoms to worsen transiently.

If, when receiving a higher concentration of oxygen, a diver's symptoms worsen, oxygen provision should normally be continued. The transient deterioration should not last for more than a few minutes unless it is caused by something other than oxygen breathing. The equipment should be checked to ensure it is functioning correctly. Things to check include the oxygen supply and the flow rate.

Chronic lung disease in the non-diving population

Some people have chronic obstructive lung disease, such as chronic bronchitis or emphysema, which may cause excess carbon dioxide to be trapped in the blood. Certain sufferers have become so accustomed to high levels of carbon dioxide that they receive their main breathing trigger from low oxygen levels, rather than from elevated carbon dioxide. On rare occassions, a sufferer of chronic obstructive lung disease may have respiratory depression or arrest when given high concentrations of oxygen. Fortunately for the diving first aider, these very sick people would be highly unlikely to be diving and would not pass a diving medical examination.

It is stressed that only a very small percentage of people react adversely to breathing elevated oxygen concentrations on the surface and they are very unlikely to be found where diving activities are being prepared or conducted. Oxygen should be provided to all divers who have respiratory distress, whose illness or injury suggests the possibility of hypoxia and to all unconscious divers. **Because the side effects of surface oxygen provision are so minimal, a trained oxygen provider should not withhold oxygen from an injured diver for fear of doing harm.**

REVIEW QUESTIONS

1. For how long can one breathe 100% oxygen at atmospheric pressure before risking pulmonary oxygen toxicity?
2. How is pulmonary oxygen toxicity prevented?
3. Beyond approximately what partial pressure of inspired oxygen may CNS oxygen toxicity occur?
4. Why may a hyperventilating diver have difficulty breathing oxygen from a demand system?

Chapter 7

STORAGE AND HANDLING OF OXYGEN

Oxygen equipment has two main components - a source of oxygen and the delivery system. There is a variety of oxygen equipment on the market, which differs to some extent from country to country. The use of most types of oxygen equipment requires advanced knowledge and skills which can be gained only through appropriate training.

Potential problems include:

- fire hazard from oxygen gas
- potential for explosion of cylinder
- improper use of certain equipment can endanger the injured person
- premature exhaustion of oxygen supply

Consequently, **it is essential for oxygen providers to be thoroughly familiar with any oxygen equipment that they may use.**

The equipment should be clean and operational and the appropriate device must be selected for the diver receiving care. The injured diver must be monitored even more closely once an oxygen delivery system, ventilation assistance device or airway management device is used. In addition, it is important that the equipment is properly discarded, cleaned or tested after use.

Resuscitation measures must never be delayed in order to locate, retrieve and assemble an oxygen delivery system. The equipment should be ready for immediate use.

OXYGEN GAS

Oxygen is produced commercially from air by a process called fractional distillation. During this process, air is initially compressed, cooled and liquified before being allowed to rewarm slowly. When the air rewarms, its various components (mainly oxygen and nitrogen) boil off when they reach their particular boiling temperature and each gas can be collected and stored under pressure in cylinders.

"The 22nd edition of the U.S. Pharmocopeia/National Formulary (USP/NF), published in 1989, states that medical grade (A) oxygen must contain a minimum of 99.0% (mole/mole) oxygen. The other 1% is usually composed of water, nitrogen, argon and other rare gases. Allowable contaminants are limited to a maximum of 300 parts per million (ppm) carbon dioxide and 10 ppm carbon monoxide. Odor must be absent during a subjective olfactory (smell) test, and foreign substances and impurities inconsistent with good pharmaceutical practice should also be absent." (Corry, 1990)

Oxygen can be a fire hazard

For a fire, four components are necessary: (1) combustible material; (2) oxygen; (3) a source of ignition; and (4) the unwise person who puts 1, 2 and 3 together!

Oxygen is a highly reactive gas which combines readily with most elements producing heat in the process. This process, known as oxidation, is one of the most common chemical reactions. In the atmosphere, steel oxidizes (rusts) but since the process is so slow we do not feel the heat that is generated. However, in a high pressure oxygen-enriched environment, steel oxidizes quickly. This is how it is cut with oxy-acetylene equipment.

Any metal or plastic can burn in oxygen given the right conditions. Oil or grease are particularly reactive with oxygen and the presence of even minute amounts of hydrocarbon oil or grease in a high pressure oxygen atmosphere can cause an explosion. If oxygen equipment is contaminated with grease, it could ignite and destroy the regulator or valve.

Leakage from a cylinder or exhaust oxygen from a person receiving oxygen first aid can very quickly produce a high oxygen content in enclosed spaces.

Since oxygen is a colorless, odorless and tasteless gas, it is difficult to detect the accumulation of elevated concentrations of oxygen. This creates a greatly increased risk of fire or explosion due to the far greater flammability of substances in this environment. Therefore, oxygen cylinders must never be stored or used in an inadequately ventilated area, or near flammable or burning substances, including cigarettes.

OXYGEN CYLINDERS

Oxygen cylinders come in a number of different sizes (Table 7.1) and should be rated by the Department of Transportation (DOT) and/or the Canadian Transportation Commission (CTC) for oxygen service. They are color-coded and, in the United States and Canada, medical oxygen cylinders are coded green. The cylinders should also be clearly labelled. The color-coding may vary from country to country. For example, in the United Kingdom, Australasia and various other places, medical oxygen cylinders are black with a white top. In Germany they are blue all over. The travelling diver should be aware of this variation. *It is important to check the label on the cylinder.*

Like SCUBA cylinders, oxygen cylinders are manufactured from either steel or aluminum alloy, and, since they hold gas under high pressure, they must be carefully handled, maintained and tested at regular intervals. As with diving cylinders, there are numerous markings on oxygen cylinders which provide information including: the serial number, date of manufacture, working pressure, capacity and test date.

"The industry standard is to perform an exterior visual inspection each time a cylinder is filled. Internal visual inspections are usually only conducted on cylinders which have been emptied during use or prior to the hydrostatic test. Aluminum cylinders require hydrostatic testing every five years and may be filled to the service pressure only. Steel cylinders also require hydrostatic testing at five year intervals and may be 10% overfilled only if a "+" (plus) symbol appears after the current hydrostatic test date. If a star symbol appears after the current hydrostatic test date on a steel cylinder, the cylinder is approved for a ten year hydrostatic test interval. Testing beyond the standard hydrostatic test is required for both the 10% overfill and ten year hydrostatic interval approvals. Additionally, for the star approval, the steel cylinder must have been hammer tested prior to every fill, filled only with oxygen at a dew point of -52°F @ 1 ATA, and never used for underwater breathing." (Corry, 1990)

Medical oxygen should not be more than 5 years old when used.

Industrial oxygen should not be substituted for medical oxygen.

When prepared, the purity of medical and industrial oxygen is identical. However, different processes are involved in filling medical and industrial oxygen cylinders and these may affect the purity of the gas actually contained in the cylinders.

A medical oxygen cylinder is completely evacuated before being refilled with pure oxygen. On the other hand, an industrial cylinder may not be evacuated prior to being refilled. It is effectively topped off. If the cylinder was drained when used (which is often the case), and, if the valve was left open, contaminants in the surrounding atmosphere may have entered the cylinder. Carbon monoxide, odors and industrial solvents are just some of the contaminants that may be present. These contaminants would normally not be removed when the cylinder is refilled and may prove toxic. Hence, *it may not be safe to breathe the gas from an industrial oxygen cylinder because the oxygen may be contaminated.* Although in an emergency, if no other oxygen source was available, industrial oxygen could probably be breathed with relative safety, this practice is not encouraged.

TABLE 7.1

Medical Oxygen Cylinder Specifications Aluminum (Luxfer USA, Ltd.)				
Type	Service Pressure (psi)	Liters	Cubic feet	E.W. w/o valve (lbs)
Medical 9	2015	249.0	8.8	3.9
D	2015	413.2	14.6	5.5
Jumbo D	2216	636.8	22.5	9.0
E	2015	682.0	24.1	8.1
M 60*	2216	1748.9	61.8	23.1
Medical M*	2216	3495.0	123.5	40.6
(Medical 9 = "C")				

TABLE 7.2

Medical Oxygen Cylinder Specifications
Steel
(Pressed Steel Tank Company)

Type	Service Pressure (psi)**	Liters **	Cubic feet**	E.W. w/o valve (lbs)
D	2015/2216	410.4/450.0	14.5/15.9	7.5
E	2015/2216	682.0/744.3	24.1/26.3	10.5
		(Norris Cylinder Company)		
M*	2015/2216	3178.1/3497.9	112.3/123.6	61.0
G*	2015/2216	6378.9/7021.2	225.4/248.1	115.0
H*	2015/2216	7148.6/7861.7	252.6/277.8	116.0
J*	2015/2216	8549.4/9387.1	302.1/331.7	140.0

* Do not accept regulators with pin-indexed yoke (CGA-870 fitting); require CGA-540 fitting.

** Secondary figures apply if cylinder is "+" rated for 10% overfill. The service pressure on both aluminum and steel cylinders is roll stamped into the shoulder of the cylinder.

Tables 7.1 and 7.2 reprinted from Corry, 1990.

Divers should ensure that there will be an adequate oxygen supply to allow an injured diver to breathe 100% oxygen from the dive site until reaching an appropriate medical facility. To ensure this, it is often advisable to use a large cylinder or a number of small cylinders.

The D, E and jumbo D cylinders are most commonly carried in the field by diving instructors and EMS personnel.

As well as having an adequate capacity, the cylinder must be compact enough to fit on the dive boat. Larger boats or permanent sites may have the potential for a large oxygen store, but consideration should be given to the possible need for the equipment to accompany an injured diver while being transported to a hospital or recompression chamber. For this reason, it may be preferable to have a number of smaller cylinders rather than just a large one. DAN has suggested a minimum two hour oxygen supply be available for treatment and transport of a dive accident victim. (Dovenbarger, 1988)

A diver's emergency plan should provide a reasonable estimate of how much oxygen would be required on site in the event of an accident. This should be based on maximizing the oxygen concentration, the location of proposed diving activities, the availability of pre-hospital emergency care and the time it is likely to take the EMS personnel to reach an injured diver.

Oxygen cylinders should not be allowed to empty below the *safe residual*. The safe residual for an oxygen cylinder is determined when the pressure gauge reads 200 psi. At this point there may not be enough oxygen in the cylinder to allow for proper delivery to the injured diver. Prior to reaching 200 psi, the cylinder should be changed and replaced with a full cylinder.

The duration of a cylinder can be estimated by using the following formula:

$$D = \frac{Vr \times GP}{Pr \times R}$$

where D = duration in minutes, Vr = rated cylinder volume in liters, Pr = rated cylinder pressure in psi, GP = gauge pressure in psi minus the safe residual, and R = constant flow rate (for constant flow devices) or minute volume (for demand systems) in liters.

FIGURE 7.1

Various sizes of medical oxygen cylinders

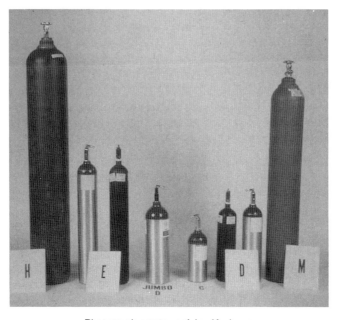

Photograph courtesy of Jon Kushner

A jumbo D cylinder should provide approximately 50 minutes of oxygen to an injured diver, with a tidal volume of 800 ml, breathing from a demand valve at a rate of 15 breaths per minute. The same cylinder would be expected to last for around 40 minutes if used with a constant flow delivery system set at 15 liters per minute (lpm). When providing emergency oxygen to divers suffering from decompression illness, DAN recommends a minimum flow rate of 15 lpm for constant flow delivery devices. However, a tight-fitting face mask with a demand valve is preferred since it delivers a higher oxygen concentration.

Larger cylinders will last proportionately longer and are desirable since divers often dive in areas remote from medical facilities.

Cylinder valves

Smaller medical oxygen cylinders (up to size E) are fitted with a pin-indexed medical oxygen valve which will only mate with the appropriate oxygen regulator (Figure 7.2). Two machined holes in the valve body index with two pins on the appropriate oxygen regulator. This system is designed to prevent an oxygen regulator being attached to a gas supply other than oxygen.

FIGURE 7.2

CGA-870 pin-indexed valve and matching regulator

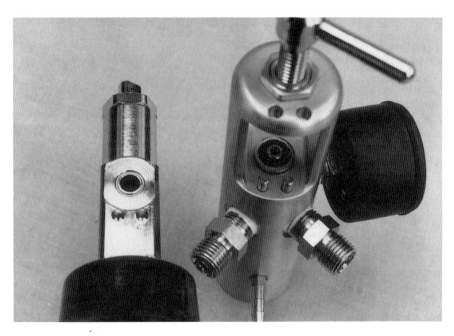

Larger medical oxygen cylinders and industrial oxygen cylinders are fitted with a threaded fitting as shown in Figure 7.3.

FIGURE 7.3

CGA-540 valve for regulators with a threaded fitting

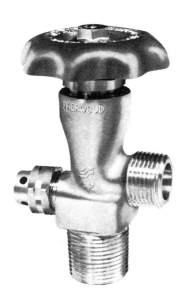

The valves on oxygen cylinders contain a fusible link which is designed to degrade in temperatures in excess of 165°F. This is to prevent the cylinder from rupturing if exposed to excessive temperatures. "This link is an additional safety feature to prevent the standard frangible disk from accidentally discharging the cylinder during critical times such as surgery, or actual emergency oxygen administration during transport." (Corry, 1990)

Adapters

Various adapters designed to permit diving regulators to be fitted to oxygen cylinders have appeared over the years. These adapters are sometimes "home-made" by people trying to economize on the purchasing of oxygen equipment.

Such devices can be hazardous since, if they are not properly designed or machined, they can cause excessive heat to be generated when oxygen flows rapidly through them. One report graphically describes the fire that resulted when a silicone-filled regulator was attached to such an adapter:

When the cylinder valve was turned on, sparks erupted from the water sensing holes in the first stage. They started like a sparkler on bonfire night and got progressively stronger like a Mount Vesuvius firecracker as the oxygen carved out parent metal. I kicked the cylinder away and a small explosion occurred. The fire abated and the cylinder valve was turned off... I have no doubt that if the regulator had been in a diver's mouth the result would have been fatal." (Walters, 1985) The adapter and damaged regulator are shown in Figures 7.4 and 7.5.

FIGURE 7.4

Home made adapter and damaged regulator resulting from an oxygen fire

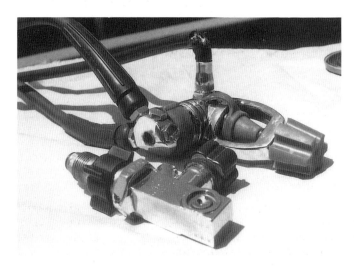

FIGURE 7.5

Damaged regulator resulting from an oxygen fire

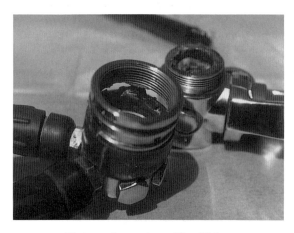

Photographs courtesy of Des Walters

Commercially-produced adapters are also available. A specially cleaned (oxygen clean) and oxygen compatible regulator should be used with such a system and dedicated to its use. Oxygen regulators that require lubrication usually use a fluorinated grease, since most lubricants are incompatible with high pressure oxygen (many are also incompatible with high pressure air). No hydrocarbon lubricant is recommended for use with oxygen. Silicone lubricants are often used in diving regulators. Dow Corning, the manufacturer of many of these silicone lubricants, has stated that its lubricants must not be used with oxygen. One lubricant, CHRISTO-LUBE MCG-111, recently developed by Lubrication Technology Inc., has proved to be compatible with both high pressure and liquid oxygen. This relatively expensive lubricant is a perfluoro-polyether grease, thickened by a powdered fluorotelemer.

Attachment of any delivery system, other than an oxygen clean, compatible and dedicated regulator and hose, is not wise and is not recommended.

REGULATORS

An oxygen regulator is a pressure reducer which reduces the cylinder pressure, of approximately 2000 to 2200 psi, to an outlet pressure compatible with the delivery equipment. A pressure or contents gauge is usually attached directly to, or on line with, the regulator. Some cylinder valves have a pressure gauge attached.

Many different types of medical oxygen regulators are available. Some provide relatively high flow rates suitable for a delivery device such as a demand valve, and/or for a suction device. Others provide lower flow rates suitable for a delivery system such as a pocket-type mask or a bag-valve resuscitator. The most versatile are capable of supplying both high and low flow rates so they can be used with a broad range of delivery systems.

"Ambu, Life Support Products, MADA Medical Products and Veriflo are the major companies in the United States manufacturing these multi-function regulators. All four manufacturers' regulators have yokes which are pin-indexed so they may only be attached to their counterpart pin-indexed oxygen valves (CGA-870) which are used with the D, E and Jumbo D cylinders. These regulators each have two male Diameter Index Safety System (DISS) outlets (approximately 50 psi) and a barbed continuous flow outlet nipple. Each DISS outlet generally has a peak flow rate of 160 lpm but may be as high as 190 to 250 lpm due to individual variations. This flow rate may be as low as 100 lpm if cylinder pressure is very low, self-sealing valves are incorporated into the outlet, or both outlets are being used to peak capacity. All four regulators should be able to supply adequate oxygen to two demand valves operating at the same time as long as the cylinder pressure is above 200 to 300 psi.

All four regulators are also available with a CGA-540 fitting instead of the yoke, for mounting on larger medical oxygen cylinders. The Ambu and Life Support Products regulators have variable constant flow capability from 0 to 25 lpm, while the MADA Medical Products and Veriflo regulators are variable from 0 to 15 lpm." (Corry, 1990)

FIGURE 7.6
Life Support Products regulator
(with variable flow of 0-25 lpm and two DISS outlets)

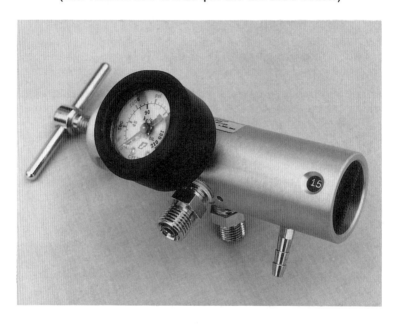

FIGURE 7.7
Ambu regulator
(with variable flow of 0-25 lpm and two DISS outlets)

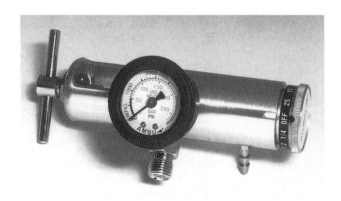

FIGURE 7.8
Veriflo (Sierra) Regulator
(with variable flow of 2-15 lpm and two DISS outlets)

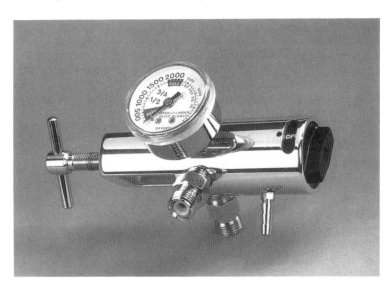

FIGURE 7.9
Life Support Products regulator with CGA-540 threaded fitting

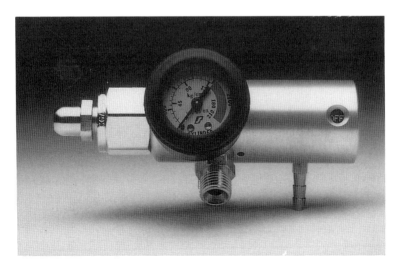

PREPARING THE OXYGEN SUPPLY

First, the valve cover is removed, if present. The valve wrench or handwheel should be fitted, if necessary. Avoid using ferrous metal wrenches with oxygen equipment since such material can produce a spark if it strikes against metal objects. Impurities are purged from the orifice of the cylinder valve before the regulator is attached to it. This process, known as *cracking* or *snifting* the valve, is done by slowly easing the valve on and closing it after having blown out any debris. The oxygen outlet should be facing down and away from the oxygen provider, and others present, during this process. After the valve is cracked, it is only lightly closed so that it can be opened easily when the regulator is attached. If the valve is obstructed and is suddenly opened, the rapid increase in pressure produces high temperatures. Fragments of foreign material such as brass filings in valves have caused cylinder fires.

It is virtually impossible to get a leakproof seal between the metal surfaces of the valve and a pin-indexed regulator without the aid of a sealing washer.

Two types of washer are available: (1) A nylon washer which is designed for single use; and (2) a Bodok seal, which is a neoprene o-ring that is held captive in an aluminum surround to prevent it distorting when under pressure. The Bodok seal can be reused until worn or damaged. Spare sealing washers should be kept with the equipment in case the one fitted is lost or damaged.

FIGURE 7.10

Bodok seal

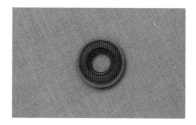

If the regulator and valve are pin-indexed, the regulator must be positioned so that the locating pins on it are lined up with the matching holes on the cylinder valve pillar. The yoke screw is then tightened firmly enough to hold the regulator in position when the valve is opened. The regulator is secured by the oxygen pressure after the valve is opened.

All the flow valves should be closed so that leaks can be detected when the valve is opened. In the event of pressure gauge failure, the face plate of the gauge could be ejected. Accordingly, the oxygen provider should ensure the pressure gauge is not facing anyone, or cover the face of the pressure gauge while the valve is being opened.

The valve should be opened slowly, so the regulator is pressurized slowly. The reading of the pressure gauge should be noted and the valve should then be closed briefly while observing the gauge. Any drop in pressure indicates a leak in the system, which should be located and rectified before proceeding.

It is generally recommended that the cylinder valve is turned on fully and then back half a turn. However, DAN recommends that the valve be slowly opened one full turn. This should provide adequate oxygen and will facilitate rapid closure and eventual removal and replacement of empty cylinders. The oxygen supply is now prepared.

Note:

The oxygen supply should always be prepared (and flowing in the case of constant flow devices) before the delivery device is placed on the diver. In addition, the supply should remain on until after the delivery device is removed from the diver.

REVIEW QUESTIONS

1. List three potential hazards associated with the use of oxygen equipment.

2. Why is it difficult to detect a build up of oxygen gas in a room?

3. How often do oxygen cylinders need to be hydrostatically tested?

4. Why may it be dangerous to breathe industrial oxygen?

5. How much oxygen should be available to treat a diver?

6. What is the approximate range of working pressures for oxygen cylinders in the United States?

7. Why should the cylinder valve be turned on slowly when oxygen equipment is attached?

8. Why may it be dangerous to use a regulator that is not oxygen clean, compatible and dedicated with oxygen?

To prepare the oxygen supply:

- Ensure the area is well ventilated and that there is nothing burning in the immediate vicinity (including cigarettes).
- Ensure that your hands are not greasy before handling the oxygen equipment.
- Remove the cover from the cylinder valve, if present.
- Ensure that the cylinder valve and regulator fitting are clean and free from any oil or grease.
- Fit the wrench or handwheel to the cylinder.
- Face the valve outlet away from yourself and others, and purge the valve by easing it on slowly and turning it off again.
- Check that the sealing washer is fitted.
- Fit the regulator to the valve and tighten it just sufficently to hold it in position. *Ensure it is secure.*
- Lay the unit down. Do not position yourself over the cylinder valve in case the regulator becomes displaced. Position yourself to the side of the cylinder.
- Close all flow valves.
- Ensure the pressure gauge is not facing anyone.
- Turn on the valve slowly and pressurize the regulator.
- Turn off the valve and observe the pressure gauge to detect leaks.
- If the system is leaking or fails to pressurize: (1) turn off cylinder valve; (2) set constant flow dial to zero; (3) check for presence of, or damage to, sealing washer and replace if necessary; (4) replace regulator and reopen the valve. If the system still fails to pressurize, change the cylinder and try again.
- If the system pressurizes appropriately, open the cylinder valve one full turn.
- Check the pressure gauge to determine how much oxygen is available.

Chapter 8

OXYGEN DELIVERY SYSTEMS

To maximize the benefits of oxygen first aid in diving accidents, 100% oxygen should be delivered.

In order to provide 100% oxygen to an injured diver, a delivery device must supply all of the diver's inspiratory requirements. In addition, air must be prevented from entering the system and diluting the inhaled oxygen and expired breath must be vented effectively to prevent rebreathing carbon dioxide.

There is an array of delivery devices designed for giving oxygen to conscious and/or unconscious persons. However, very little oxygen equipment has been designed specifically for treating diving accidents.

A number of available oxygen delivery systems will be reviewed in the following section and their suitability for treating an injured diver will be discussed.

It must be emphasized that the oxygen concentrations achievable using different delivery devices vary from one report to another. The oxygen concentrations quoted here are sometimes taken from manufacturers' literature and are often the maximum possible. Oxygen concentrations quoted are only those delivered at the mask. The percentage obtained by an injured person is almost impossible to measure, and is affected by breathing rate, tidal volume, supplied flow rate, volume of supply equipment and many other factors. The oxygen concentration actually achieved when some of this equipment is used in the field, and/or by an operator who is unfamiliar with it, is likely to be substantially lower than that quoted.

Masks

There are a number of different masks available which come in a variety of shapes and sizes to suit different people. Because oxygen masks cover the mouth and nose, they are referred to as oronasal masks. Some are designed to have a low volume in order to minimize dead space.

Masks are usually made from soft or hard plastic, silicone or rubber. Most masks are transparent, so the oxygen provider can more easily see if the injured diver regurgitates or vomits. In addition, with a clear mask it is possible to observe the diver's face and lip color and to see if spontaneous breathing is occurring by checking if the interior of the mask is temporarily fogging up after exhalation. Some anesthetic masks are malleable and are made from black rubber with a lead insert which allows the mask to be molded to fit the contours of the face.

The concentration of oxygen received by an injured diver via the various masks depends on how well the mask seals, the oxygen flow rate, the tidal volume and breathing rate of the diver, whether or not a reservoir bag is used in conjunction with the mask and the volume of that reservoir bag.

Tight-sealing masks

Tight-sealing masks have a sealing cuff to facilitate an effective seal. Many of the newer masks are made from PVC or silicone, and, since the cuff is relatively soft it can mold to the diver's face quite effectively. Some masks have a double seal which can be very effective.

One such mask, commonly available in the United States, is the *Tru-Fit™* mask. This mask is quite pliable and seals on a variety of faces. Since it is clear, it provides good viewing of the injured diver's face and it incorporates a chin cup to facilitate correct placement.

It has been reported that the Tru-Fit™ mask can become very stiff in cold temperatures. This appears to be the case with the mask made from PVC, but should not occur with the silicone version. PVC can relatively easily lose its original shape if left distorted for a period of time. Silicone, on the other hand, will readily return to its original form.

Other masks have rubber cuffs that require inflation prior to use. These cuffs deteriorate easily and must be checked regularly since the mask will not seal unless the cuff is adequately inflated. The cuff should be partly inflated when stored to prevent its sides from binding together. Although the cuff is designed for ambient inflation, some users prefer to inflate it a little more to facilitate a better seal. Certain other masks have a silicone cuff which is permanently inflated. These cuffs should also be checked periodically. Laerdal manufacture a mask made from clear, hard plastic with a replacable silicone sealing edge.

A tight-sealing mask will minimize air dilution. However, when a tight sealing mask is used with a constant flow delivery system (described later), if the flow rate is too low, carbon dioxide can build up in the mask, causing the injured person to breathe more rapidly (hyperventilate) and greatly reducing the potential oxygen concentration. High flow rates will minimize carbon dioxide retention but will also use up the oxygen supply more rapidly. The oxygen concentration will fall if the injured diver's breathing rate and volume increase.

Tight-sealing masks can be used to deliver oxygen to a breathing diver and for providing a barrier and seal when resuscitating a non-breathing diver. A first aider can perform rescue breathing through the mask or can use equipment to provide the inflations. In either case, a good seal needs to be obtained. Using a mask for rescue breathing eliminates the need to pinch the injured diver's nose and, in so doing, may provide a better airway for ventilating the diver. It is also aesthetically preferable. Most medical masks are fitted with a standard 15 mm/ 22 mm female coupling which can be attached to a demand valve and/or resuscitation device.

FIGURE 8.1
Various tight-sealing oxygen masks

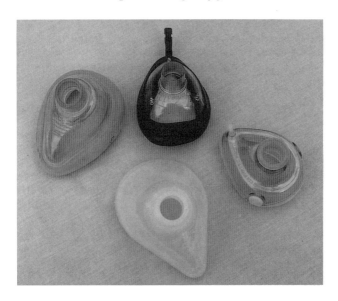

FIGURE 8.2
Mouth-to-mask resuscitation using an LSP mouth-to-mask resuscitator

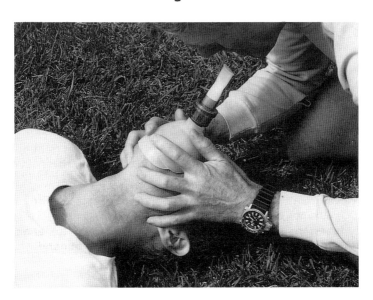

To perform mouth-to-mask resuscitation:

- Place the injured diver on the back.
- Wipe the diver's face and lips dry.
- Attach the one-way valve to the mask, if present.
- Place the mask over the diver's nose and mouth with the narrow end over the nose. Wriggle it around until it seats nicely, ensuring the best seal possible.
- Position yourself above the supine diver's head. (Alternatively, you can position yourself beside the diver, if preferred.)
- Open the airway using head tilt and jaw thrust while holding the mask to the injured diver's face.
- Use the thumb and index finger of each hand to hold the mask onto the injured diver's face while lifting the jaw from both sides with the other three fingers.
- Seal your lips around the port of the mask and blow gently. Blow sufficiently to cause the diver's lower chest and abdomen to rise. Stop blowing as soon as the chest rises.
- Ensure that the chest falls completely before ventilating again.
- Carefully monitor the diver's condition by checking the pulse and color, and act accordingly.
- Never leave the injured diver unattended.

DEMAND SYSTEMS

The easiest and most effective way to achieve near 100% oxygen with a spontaneously breathing diver is with a demand valve delivery system.

The equipment necessary to deliver oxygen in this manner is very similar in principle to SCUBA equipment. The high pressure oxygen is delivered from the cylinder through a pressure regulator (first stage) which reduces the cylinder pressure to a line (intermediate) pressure suitable for the second stage. The second stage, which incorporates a demand valve, further reduces the line pressure to ambient pressure. When a spontaneously breathing diver inhales, the demand valve opens and allows oxygen to flow through.

A demand valve with a tight-sealing, double-seal, oronasal mask is capable of delivering 100% oxygen to both the conscious and unconscious (breathing) diver (Figure 8.3). However, it is often difficult to get an adequate seal, especially if the oxygen provider is unfamiliar with, or out of practice with, the equipment. If the seal is inadequate, the oxygen concentration can fall well below the desired 100%. In addition, *the demand valve may not function effectively if the seal is inadequate since there may be insufficient suction to trigger the demand valve.*

FIGURE 8.3
A demand valve oxygen delivery system with tight-sealing mask

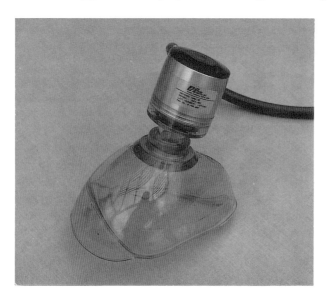

FIGURE 8.4
A demand valve oxygen delivery system utilizing a mouthpiece and nose clip

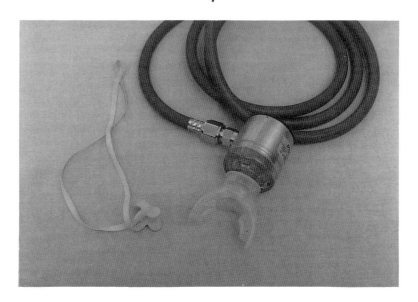

Because tight-fitting masks are sometimes uncomfortable, and because of the difficulty in achieving an adequate seal with certain masks and on some diver's faces, some demand valves can be adapted to suit a *conscious* diver by replacing the mask with a regulator mouthpiece and sealing the diver's nose with a nose clip, fingers or a diver's facemask. If the nose is not sealed, the oxygen concentration may drop well below 100% (Figure 8.4). A system fitted with a mouthpiece is not suitable for an unconscious diver since it is very difficult to get an adequate mouth seal.

Certain demand systems may require more breathing effort to open the valve than some unconscious persons can provide. This is often the case with equipment that was not specifically designed to provide oxygen to an unconscious person. Some divers have adapted SCUBA demand valves and many of these require substantial inhalation effort.

CAUTION: SCUBA equipment should not be used to provide oxygen. Only appropriate oxygen clean and compatible equipment should be used.

Two medical oxygen demand valves, the *Elder* and *LSP* demand valves, have been commonly available in the United States. Both are manufactured by LIfe Support Products Inc. In addition, LSP Inc. distributes another demand valve known as the *LSP Bag Refill-Valve*, and has relatively recently developed a new oxygen-powered hand-held ventilator which incorporates a demand valve. This new ventilator called the *MTV*.

Some demand valves are only suitable for breathing divers. These are known as **demand inhalator valves**, and include the *LSP* demand inhalator valve and the *LSP Bag Refill-Valve.*

Other demand valves incorporate a button or trigger to facilitate ventilation of a non-breathing diver. Such devices are known as **manually triggered oxygen-powered resuscitators** or **CPR/Demand Valves**. These include the *LSP* and *Elder* CPR/Demand Valves as well as the *MTV*.

LSP Demand Inhalator Valve and CPR/Demand Valve

The body of the LSP demand valve is made from anodized aluminum with a polysulfone outlet adapter and a polycarbonate cover. It is designed to operate with a regulated oxygen supply of around 40 to 90 psi at temperatures from approximately -30°F to 125°F. Its "crack" pressure is 0 to -2 cmH$_2$O with an exhalation resistance from 1.5 to 6.4 cmH$_2$O, depending on the flow rate. It is available with a flow rate set at either 40 or 160 lpm at 50 psi and a delivery pressure of 60 $\pm$ 5 cmH$_2$O. The valve is available with or without a positive pressure button. The LSP demand inhalator valve (Figure 8.3) is currently incorporated in the oxygen unit distributed to divers by DAN.

FIGURE 8.5

LSP CPR/Demand valve

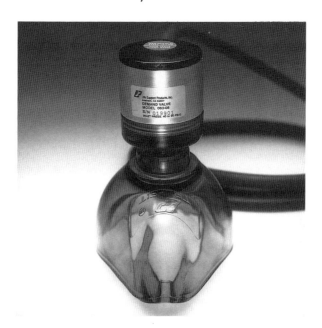

The Elder CPR/Demand Valve

The Elder CPR/Demand Valve is also manufactured by Life Support Products Inc. The valve body is made from high impact plastic and the moving and adjustable parts from stainless steel. It is designed to operate with a regulated oxygen supply of around 40 to 90 psi at temperatures from approximately -30°F to 125°F. Its specified "crack" pressure is 0 to - 2.5 cmH2O with a delivery pressure of 60 ± 5 cmH2O unless otherwise indicated. It is available with a flow rate set at either 40 or 160 lpm at 50 psi for both resuscitation and demand modes.

LSP Bag Refill-Valve

The body of the Bag Refill-Valve is made from high impact polyester with the moving and adjusting parts being made from stainless steel. This valve is designed to function with any oxygen system with an outlet pressure of 40 to 90 psi and a flow rate of around 160 to 200 lpm, at temperatures from -40°F to 140°F. Its specifications state that it can provide a flow rate of around 200 lpm at 50 psi supply pressure. However, this depends on a number of factors, which include the pressure regulator it is used with. (Generally, the maximum flow of the demand valve is equal to the unimpeded flow from the supply source less about 30%). The LSP Bag Refill-Valve demand inhalator valve is specified as requiring an inspiratory effort of -0.5 cmH$_2$O to open the valve.

FIGURE 8.6
Elder CPR/Demand valve

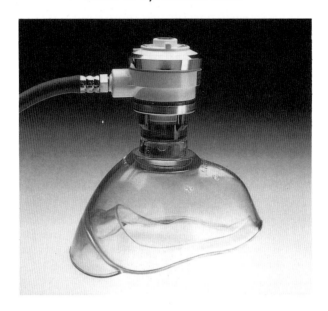

FIGURE 8.7
LSP Bag Refill-Valve

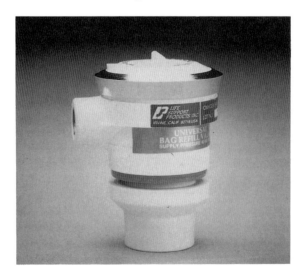

MTV

As mentioned previously, LSP Inc. has developed a new hand-held ventilator, known as the MTV, which incorporates a demand valve.

The MTV is designed to have a "crack" pressure of -1.0 to -2.5 cmH_2O. Once the flow has been triggered, a pneumatic control circuit matches the person's inspiratory demands and will deliver a flow rate up to about 100 lpm to a spontaneously breathing person.

When the ventilation button is triggered, the MTV is designed to provide a fixed flow rate of 40 lpm. Whereas other manually triggered oxygen-powered resuscitators are designed to terminate oxygen flow when a back pressure of around 60 cmH_2O is detected, the MTV will terminate both flow and pressure. Both flow and pressure are vented to the atmosphere, and the pressure should immediately return to baseline pressure, so avoiding the risk of damaging the injured person's lungs. A secondary relief valve, set at about 70 cmH_2O, is incorporated in case the primary valve fails to relieve the pressure at its prescribed limit.

FIGURE 8.8

MTV

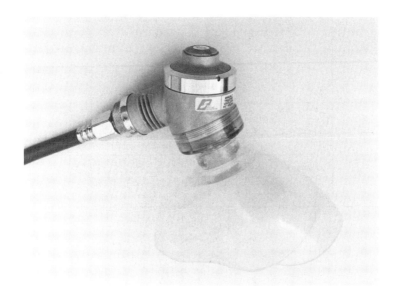

The mask adapters on all the demand valves described have a 22 mm outside diameter and 15 mm inside diameter and will fit standard medical oxygen masks.

The specifications quoted above were provided by the manufacturer. Devices in the field must be tested on a regular basis, and seviced as appropriate, to ensure that they meet the manufacturer's specifications.

Table 8.1 shows the results of some preliminary tests conducted to measure the breathing resistance of the LSP, Elder and Bag Refill oxygen demand valves, as well as the MTV. One of each type of valve was obtained from its Australian distributor. The measurements were made using a Magnehelic, manufactured by Dwyer Industries.

The first result corresponds to quiet breathing (14 per minute) and the second (in brackets) corresponds to rapid breathing (50 per minute).

TABLE 8.1

Breathing resistance (cmH_2O) of various demand valves			
Unit	Cracking Pressure	Inhalation Resistance	Exhalation Resistance
Elder	0.5 (0.5)	1.5 (2.5)	1.0 (2.5)
LSP	2.5 (2.5)	2.5 (2.0)	1.5 (2.0)
Bag Refill	0.5 (1.0)	0.5 (2.0)	1.5 (2.0)
MTV	2.5 (3.0)	3.0 (3.0)	1.8 (2.0)

USING A DEMAND DELIVERY SYSTEM

Conscious diver

As mentioned previously, most divers requiring oxygen provision will be conscious. In the United States, the oxygen provider must obtain permission from the injured diver before providing oxygen. An oxygen provider is advised to say something to the effect of: *"This is oxygen. It will make you feel better. May I help you?"* For unconscious injured divers, permission is assumed.

When using a demand valve system with a conscious diver:

- Reassure the injured diver, explain what you are doing and ask permission to provide oxygen.
- Position the diver appropriately. If decompression illness is suspected, the diver should be laid down flat. Heart attack sufferers may prefer to be sitting or semi-reclined as they are often less breathless in this position.
- Ensure the area is well ventilated and that there is nothing burning in the immediate vicinity.
- Prepare the oxygen supply.
- If using a mask, attach the mask to the outlet adapter on the demand valve and breathe from it to ensure that it is performing adequately and to reassure the injured diver.
- If using a mask, position it carefully over the diver's nose and mouth with the narrow end over the nose. Ensure the best seal possible. Encouraging the diver to hold the mask themself may provide some reassurance.
- If using a system with a mouthpiece, ensure that the injured diver's lips form a seal around the mouthpiece. Also ensure that the diver's nose is sealed off by a nose clip or some other means.
- Ask the diver to breathe slowly and deeply. If the demand valve is not triggering, ask the diver to breathe a little more deeply to trigger the valve.
- Record the periods of oxygen breathing and the diver's response.
- Carefully monitor the diver's condition and never leave them unattended.
- Carefully monitor the oxygen supply and remove the mask or mouthpiece immediately if the supply becomes exhausted, or the diver complains that they "can't breathe". Recheck the apparatus.

Unconscious spontaneously breathing diver

When using a demand valve system with an unconscious, breathing diver:

- Place the diver in the recovery position, ensure the airway is clear, and open the airway by head tilt and chin lift.
- Ensure the area is well ventilated and that there is nothing burning in the immediate vicinity.
- Prepare the oxygen supply.
- Attach the mask to the outlet adapter of the demand valve and breathe from it to ensure it is performing adequately.
- Position the mask carefully over the diver's nose and mouth with the narrow end over the nose. Ensure the best seal possible or the demand valve may not function effectively. Some masks can be secured by a head harness.
- Record the periods of oxygen breathing and the diver's response.
- Carefully monitor the injured diver's condition by checking the airway, breathing, pulse and color.
- If the diver is having difficulty triggering the demand valve, remove it and use a constant flow delivery device instead.
- Carefully monitor the oxygen supply and remove the mask immediately if the supply becomes exhausted.
- Never leave the injured diver unattended.

FIGURE 8.9
A conscious diver breathing from a demand valve

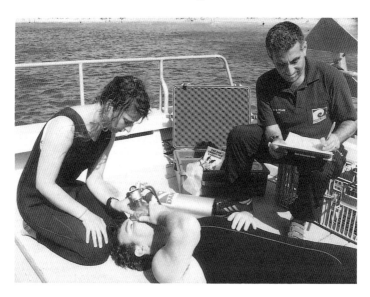

FIGURE 8.10
An unconscious diver breathing from a demand valve

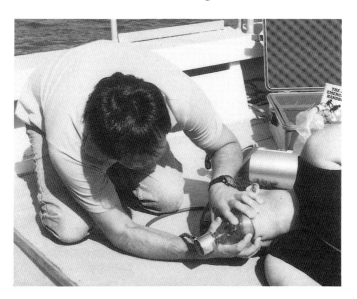

A demand inhalator system (one which is not fitted with a positive pressure ventilation button) can also be used to provide an elevated oxygen concentration to an unconscious, non-breathing diver. The first aider breathes the oxygen from the demand valve themself (with their nose sealed) and then exhales the expired breath into the non-breathing diver. This procedure may prove useful if the demand inhalator valve is the only oxygen delivery system available. However, oxygen providers are encouraged to have both demand and constant flow delivery systems to enable them to cope with a variety of emergency situations.

Unconscious non-breathing diver

When using a demand inhalator system with an unconscious diver who is not breathing:

- Clear the diver's airway.
- Position the injured diver flat on the back.
- Open the airway using maximum head tilt and chin lift.
- Commence rescue breathing immediately and continue while the oxygen equipment is being prepared by another first aider. Check the carotid pulse.
- Ensure the area is well ventilated and that there is nothing burning in the immediate vicinity.
- Prepare the oxygen supply.
- Breathe from the demand valve to ensure it is performing adequately.
- Take a breath of 100% oxygen from the demand valve (ensuring that your nose is sealed if using a system fitted with a mouthpiece), and exhale your expired breath into the injured diver. Continue ventilating the diver in this manner, as appropriate.
- Carefully monitor the diver's condition by checking the airway, breathing, pulse and color.
- Never leave the injured diver unattended.

FIGURE 8.11

Commence rescue breathing immediately and continue while the oxygen equipment is being prepared

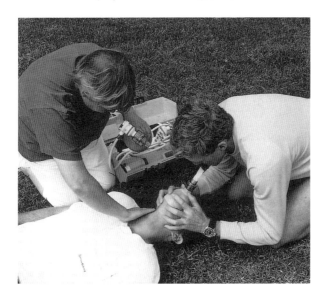

MANUALLY TRIGGERED OXYGEN-POWERED RESUSCITATORS

Manually triggered oxygen-powered resuscitators must only be used by appropriately trained and experienced operators. They must not be used on infants and children. Such devices are not recommended by DAN for use by the individual without appropriate training.

Manually triggered oxygen-powered devices (CPR/Demand valves) permit positive pressure to be initiated or terminated instantaneously by the touch of a trigger. When the trigger is fully depressed, flow rates in excess of 160 lpm of oxygen may be delivered by certain devices, although the more modern devices generally deliver flow rates up to 40 lpm.

As mentioned earlier, the Elder and LSP CPR/Demand valves are available with the flow rate set at either 40 lpm or 160 lpm for both demand and resuscitation modes. The MTV provides flow rates up to 100 lpm in demand mode, but is limited to 40 lpm in resuscitation mode.

When used for resuscitation, high flow devices are easily capable of inflating the stomach and causing regurgitation. In addition, most of these devices may have the potential to generate enough pressure to cause pulmonary barotrauma. However, a well trained and practised operator can limit the flow by pressing the trigger briefly and lightly, or by pressing only on the edge (rather than the center) of the resuscitation button.

A pressure relief valve is fitted to these devices to prevent pressures exceeding the designed outlet pressure. Oxygen flow is terminated when a back pressure greater than about 60 cmH_2O is detected. Most units terminate flow but do not release the pressure. The MTV terminates both flow and pressure and vents to the atmosphere to avoid the risk of damaging the injured person's lungs.

The relief valve should prevent lung injury to an adult but will not prevent stomach inflation which normally occurs at esophageal pressures greater than about 20 cmH_2O. Most of the devices may cease to deliver gas flow prematurely without alerting the operator. This is likely to occur in persons with high airway resistance or poor lung compliance, or both. Some devices can be fitted with an audible alarm to alert the operator to high airway pressures.

Manually triggered oxygen-powered resuscitators should provide:

"(1) a constant flow rate of 100% oxygen at less than 40 lpm (for positive pressure ventilation); (2) an inspiratory pressure relief valve that opens at approximately 60 cmH_2O and vents any remaining volume to the atmosphere or ceases gas flow; the valve may be set to 80 cmH_2O when used by advanced rescuers but only under medical direction; (3) an audible alarm that sounds whenever the relief valve pressure is exceeded to alert the rescuer that the victim requires high inflation pressures and may not be receiving adequate ventilatory volumes; (4) satisfactory operation under common environmental conditions and extremes of temperature; and (5) a demand flow system that does not impose additional work. Many oxygen-powered breathing devices currently available have restricted flow rates of 40 lpm and require unacceptably high triggering pressures in the demand mode and should not be used for spontaneously breathing patients.

Oxygen-powered devices should have the following minimum design features: (1) a standard 15 mm/22 mm coupling for mask, endotracheal tube, esophageal obturator airway, tracheostomy tube, and other alternative invasive airways; (2) a rugged, breakage-resistant mechanical design that is compact and easy to hold; and (3) a trigger positioned so that both hands of the rescuer can remain on the mask to hold it in position." (JAMA, 1992)

Oxygen-powered ventilators have several disadvantages. First and foremost, they are dependent on an oxygen supply and become useless once the supply is depleted. Unless the unit is fitted with an audible warning, an operator may not feel resistance during inflation and, therefore, may not easily detect an airway blockage or lung overpressure. (However, it has been argued that regular users can develop a feel for lung compliance by observing chest movement and demand valve sounds.) The pressures generated can cause stomach inflation and regurgitation. In addition, if a safety valve is not fitted or functioning correctly, or if the device is used on a very small person, lung damage may occur. The MTV is designed to address some of these problems.

Advantages of CPR/Demand valves include less operator fatigue, higher volumes to compensate for leaks and higher potential oxygen concentrations. Such devices can be very effective in trained skilled hands. However, they may be dangerous when used incorrectly.

FIGURE 8.12
Ventilating a non-breathing person using an Elder CPR/Demand Valve

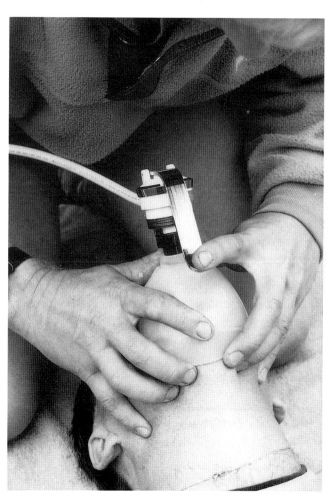

WARNING:

It requires special skills to ventilate a person with a manually triggered oxygen-powered resuscitator. These skills can only be gained through appropriate training and adequate practice. Such devices should never be used by those not trained to do so since they carry a high potential for stomach inflation and regurgitation and may also cause lung rupture.

When ventilating a diver using a manually triggered oxygen-powered resuscitator:

- Position the injured diver flat on the back.
- Commence rescue breathing immediately and continue while the oxygen equipment is being prepared by another oxygen provider.
- Ensure the area is well ventilated and that there is nothing burning in the immediate vicinity.
- Prepare the oxygen supply.
- Check the safety valve to ensure it is working. Block off the outlet with one hand and trigger the device. Oxygen flow should cease.
- Attach the mask securely.
- Place the mask over the diver's nose and mouth with the narrow end over the nose, ensuring the best seal possible.
- Position yourself behind the diver's head. Open the airway using head tilt and jaw thrust while holding the mask to the diver's face.
- Ventilate the diver by carefully squeezing the trigger (or pressing the button), while watching the diver's chest, and releasing it relatively quickly. Ventilate just enough to cause the lower chest and abdomen to rise. *Release the trigger/button as soon as the chest begins to rise.*
- Observe the stomach for distension and watch for regurgitation.
- Continue to ventilate the injured diver at the appropriate rate.
- Monitor the diver's color and pulse and act accordingly.
- Never leave the injured diver unattended.

Note:

If you are unable to ventilate the diver effectively using the oxygen resuscitator, revert to rescue breathing.

CONSTANT FLOW SYSTEMS

The most commonly available oxygen systems are those that provide a constant flow of oxygen. These systems still utilize an oxygen regulator to reduce the cylinder pressure. However, instead of using a demand valve, which supplies oxygen only on demand, they provide a constant flow of oxygen at either a fixed or adjustable flow rate.

Constant flow systems usually cannot deliver the high oxygen concentrations achievable with demand systems. Because high flow rates are required to achieve high oxygen concentrations with constant flow systems, delivery time can be greatly reduced if the oxygen supply is limited.

A fixed flow rate is achieved by means of a flow restrictor, which is a barbed outlet or nipple with an orifice of a predetermined size. However, most systems available in the United States incorporate variable flow meters, which usually provide flow rates of around 0 to 15 lpm or 0 to 25 lpm.

Some variable flow meters have a gauge with a needle to indicate the rate (Figure 8.13), while others utilize a marked dial or window by which to set the tap, rather than a gauge (Figure 8.14).

FIGURE 8.13

Western Enterprises regulator with variable flow meter

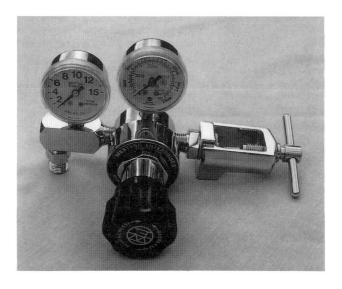

FIGURE 8.14

LSP regulator with variable flow rate indicated within the window

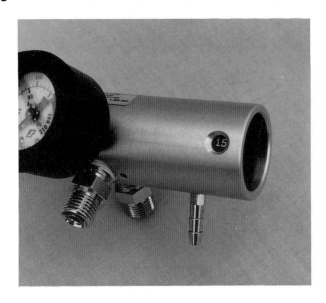

Another type of variable flow meter, sometimes called the *Thorpe Tube*, consists of a clear acrylic tube with a small metal ball inside. Oxygen flows into the tube and lifts the ball. The flow rate is adjusted by turning the tap and the resultant flow rate is read from the top of the ball. Since this meter must be used in an upright position, it sometimes creates problems during diver transport. It is also relatively fragile and may be damaged during field use.

Oxygen is usually transferred from the regulator to a constant flow delivery device via tubing. Translucent PVC oxygen supply tubing (usually with an internal diameter of around 4.8 mm) is attached to the barbed outlet, the other end being attached to the delivery system. The tubing is simply pushed onto the barbed outlet until it is secure.

DELIVERY DEVICES USED WITH CONSTANT FLOW SYSTEMS

The oxygen concentration delivered by a constant flow system depends on the oxygen flow rate, the type of delivery system (e.g. type of mask), the effectiveness of the seal and the rate and depth of the injured diver's breathing. In almost all cases the oxygen concentration will be well below 100%. It varies from about 24 to 60% with a nasal cannula or simple face mask, to near 100% with a tight-sealing bag-valve-mask system with an additional oxygen reservoir bag attached and a flow rate approaching 15 lpm.

There is a simple rule that is sometimes used to estimate the percentage oxygen being deilvered to the injured person by a constant flow delivery device:
For every one liter per minute increase in oxygen flow, you deliver approximately a 4% increase in the concentration of oxygen. However, this rule is not always reliable since many factors influence the oxygen concentration achieved.

Although most of these systems do not normally provide the maximum benefit, especially for a victim of decompression illness, they may be easier to use than tight-fitting masks and are certainly better than nothing. In addition, they may be valuable in the first aid for injuries such as shock, asthma and smoke inhalation in which 100% inspired oxygen may not be necessary, as well as for supplementing the oxygen supply during resuscitation.

Nasal cannula

A nasal cannula consists of two soft nasal prongs which are inserted into the nostrils. It is a simple, comfortable means of providing supplemental oxygen. A conscious person can talk, drink and cough without interrupting oxygen provision.

FIGURE 8.15

Nasal cannula

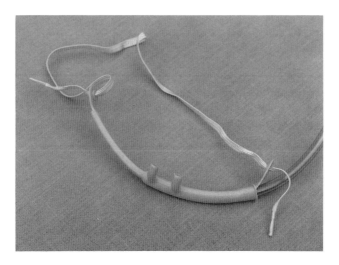

Although it can be very effective in treating many conditions requiring elevated oxygen concentrations, *a nasal cannula is far from ideal for treating decompression illness since the concentration of inspired oxygen is relatively unpredictable and is substantially lower than 100%.*

It has been reported that a nasal cannula, correctly positioned, can deliver oxygen concentrations of around 24 to 44% with flow rates of 1 to 6 lpm in a spontaneously breathing person, depending upon how much the person breathes through the mouth, among other factors. However, it is difficult to determine the oxygen concentration received by a person when using such a device. If placed far enough into the nose, a nasal cannula creates a pool of oxygen in the pharynx. When the person breathes via either mouth or nose, this pool of almost pure oxygen is the first gas to be taken into the trachea, down to the lungs and to the alveoli. The amount of oxygen reaching the alveoli depends on the rate and depth of respiration, the length of time for which the pool of oxygen has been accumulating and the volume of the nasopharynx. At a flow rate of 6 lpm the nasopharynx is filled, so increasing the flow rate will not raise the oxygen concentration appreciably. Flow rates higher than about 5 lpm are uncomfortable for the injured person as they dry out and cause trauma to the nasal mucosa, and may cause nosebleeds or headaches. Effectiveness is reduced if the person has nasal obstruction due to a cold, injury or anatomical deformity.

A nasal cannula can be used to significantly increase the oxygen level in resuscitation by inserting the prongs in the nose of either the injured person or first aider while performing rescue breathing. Using a nasal cannula with an oxygen flow rate of 3 lpm has been shown to be sufficient to cause an increase of up to 85% in arterial blood oxygen levels. Higher flow rates did not increase oxygen levels and used up the oxygen supply more quickly.

A nasal cannula should be disposed of after being used.

To use a nasal cannula:

- Position the injured diver appropriately.
- Ensure the area is well ventilated and that there is nothing burning in the immediate vicinity.
- Prepare the oxygen supply.
- Set the flow rate to 3 to 5 lpm.
- If the injured diver is conscious, reassure them. Ask permission to provide oxygen, explain what you are doing and that the hissing sound is oxygen flowing from the prongs.
- Insert the two nasal prongs into the nostrils.
- Place the supporting band around the head and tighten until secure.
- If the injured diver is conscious, ask them to breathe deeply and slowly.
- Record the periods of oxygen breathing and the diver's response.
- Carefully monitor the diver's condition by checking the airway, breathing, pulse and color, and act accordingly.
- Carefully monitor the oxygen supply and remove the cannula immediately if the supply becomes exhausted.
- Never leave the injured diver unattended.

Single nasal catheters are sometimes used by certain medical personnel to provide elevated concentrations of oxygen to an injured person. However, as with a nasal cannula, low flow rates must be used. These devices are also unsuitable for treating most diving injuries.

Simple face mask

This mask is probably the most commonly available oxygen mask. *It cannot be used on a non-breathing person.*

Because it distorts easily and has a relatively narrow sealing surface, the simple face mask often seals poorly. In addition, large ventilation holes allow the oxygen to be further diluted with air. A simple face mask is reportedly capable of delivering oxygen concentrations of 35 to 60% at flow rates from 6 to 14 lpm. Flow rates lower than 6 lpm allow excessive carbon dioxide retention since the injured person's expired breath is not flushed from the mask adequately.

FIGURE 8.16

Simple face mask

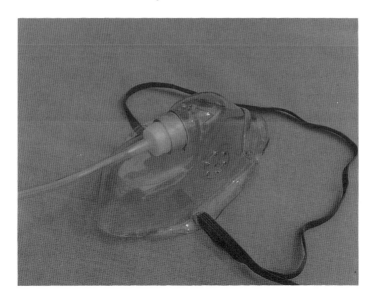

Simple face masks are far from ideal for providing oxygen to a diver suffering from decompression illness since the injured diver would still be breathing a substantial amount of nitrogen from the air entering the mask. However, they are certainly better than nothing and are very useful for treating many other ailments where an increased oxygen concentration is beneficial. Such masks can only be used for a spontaneously breathing person and cannot be used with a non-breathing person.

When using a simple face mask, ensure it fits snugly by squeezing the soft metal band against the shape of the nose. This will contribute to a higher inspired oxygen concentration and helps prevent oxygen from blowing directly into the person's eyes and causing irritation. The mask is designed to be disposable and should be discarded after use.

Some masks, known as **venturi masks**, are fitted with a venturi system which ensures that a certain flow of oxygen mixes with a certain amount of air, so providing, quite accurately, a specified concentration of oxygen (24 to 40%). The required flow rates and the corresponding oxygen concentrations should be marked on the mask. Some of these masks are designed for use by people with chronic obstructive lung disease and ensure that a fixed, relatively low oxygen percentage is delivered. Venturi masks are not suitable for diving accidents.

FIGURE 8.17

Venturi mask

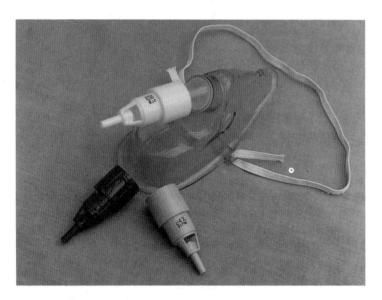

Another type of constant flow mask is fitted with a reservoir bag so that when the injured person inhales, much of the inhaled gas comes from the reservoir, thereby increasing the oxygen concentration. This is known as a **partial rebreather mask**. These masks can reportedly deliver oxygen concentrations from 35% at 6 lpm to 60% at a flow rate of 10 lpm.

Non-rebreather mask

A non-rebreather mask is fitted with both a 750 ml reservoir bag and one-way valves. This type of mask is designed to reduce the amount of air and carbon dioxide inhaled, thereby increasing the concentration of oxygen. The reservoir bag fills with oxygen and, when the injured diver inhales, a one-way valve ensures that primarily oxygen is breathed from the reservoir. When the diver exhales, the one-way valve system prevents exhaled gas from entering the reservoir. Other one-way exhaust valves cover either one or both sets of holes in the mask to prevent or minimize air entry. If valves cover both sets of holes, the injured diver cannot breathe unless there is an adequate flow of oxygen. This potential problem is overcome in those masks with a one-way valve fitted to only one set of holes, or by ensuring the injured diver is constantly monitored.

FIGURE 8.18

Non-rebreather mask

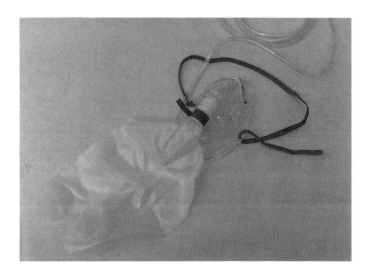

For proper use, the reservoir bag must be primed and should always contain enough oxygen so that it does not deflate fully (ideally, no more than one third) when the injured diver takes their deepest inhalation. In addition, all three one-way valves should be fitted and seating properly. A good seal also needs to be achieved. Under these ideal circumstances, a non-rebreather mask is reported to be capable of supplying an oxygen concentration of up to 95% with a flow rate of 10 to 15 lpm. However, in practice such a high concentration may be difficult to achieve and the mask will generally deliver a substantially lower oxygen concentration. A flow rate of around 25 lpm may be required to achieve an oxygen concentration near 90%. A minimum flow rate of 15 lpm is recommended when using a non-rebreather mask.

If using a non-rebreather mask, it is important to ensure the reservoir is distended with oxygen before the mask is fitted to the injured diver. To maximize the oxygen concentration, the oxygen flow rate should be adjusted so as not to allow the reservoir to deflate completely.

Although a non-rebreather mask is not capable of supplying as high oxygen concentrations as a demand system with tight-sealing mask, it can be very useful if a diver has difficulty with, or cannot use, a demand system.

FIGURE 8.19

Priming a non-rebreather mask

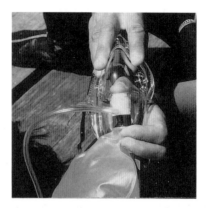

With the oxygen flowing, place your thumb over the flapper valve until the reservoir inflates.

FIGURE 8.20

Diver wearing a non-rebreather mask

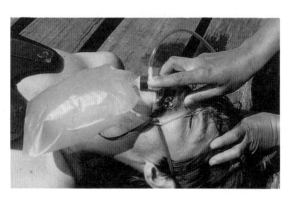

Sqeeze the metal band against the shape of the nose, ensure the mask fits as snugly as possible and that the reservoir never deflates.

When using a simple face mask or non-rebreather mask:

- Ensure the injured diver is breathing adequately.
- Position the diver appropriately. An unconscious, breathing diver should be placed in the recovery position. A conscious diver suffering from an asthma attack or heart attack may find it easier to breathe if sitting or semi-reclined.
- Ensure the area is well ventilated and that there is nothing burning in the immediate vicinity.
- Prepare the oxygen supply.
- Set the flow rate. The rate used will depend on the mask, the oxygen concentration required and the supply available. Remember that if the diver seems to be suffering from decompression illness it is better to give a high concentration as soon as possible and to continue until the supply is exhausted. The flow rate used with a non-rebreather mask should be at least 15 lpm.
- Reassure a conscious diver, ask permission to provide oxygen, explain what you are doing and that the hissing sound is oxygen flowing into the mask. Listen to the mask yourself to confirm oxygen flow, prior to placing it on the diver's face.
- If using a non-rebreather mask, ensure the reservoir is distended with oxygen before it is placed on the injured diver's face.
- Ask a conscious diver to place the mask over the mouth and nose with the narrow end upwards and the metal band (if fitted) over the bridge of the nose.
- Ask the injured diver to take deep, slow breaths.
- Position the supporting band around the diver's head and tighten until secure. Gently squeeze the metal band so that it fits snugly onto the nose. Take care not to injure an unconscious diver's eyes with the band.
- If using a non-rebreather mask, adjust the flow rate to prevent the reservoir deflating completely.
- Record the periods of oxygen breathing and the diver's response.
- Carefully monitor the injured diver's condition by checking the airway, breathing, pulse and color, and act accordingly.
- Carefully monitor the oxygen supply and remove the mask immediately if the supply becomes exhausted.
- Never leave the injured diver unattended.

Pocket-style masks

There are several different manufacturers and types of pocket-style masks. One such mask that is commonly available is the Laerdal Pocket Mask™. These masks are compact and collapsible and are therefore easily stored. Because the masks are relatively sturdy and have an effective sealing cuff, they are capable of providing an air tight seal. These masks are designed for use with rescue breathing in situations when mouth-to-mouth or mouth-to-nose contact may not be acceptable due to facial injuries, poisons or risk of infectious disease. A one-way valve can also be attached to direct the injured diver's exhaled breath away from the area of contact with the first aider's mouth. Although this is supposed to further reduce the risks of cross-infection, there is currently no evidence that it is an effective or necessary addition. It is also capable of malfunctioning.

FIGURE 8.21
Laerdal Pocket Mask™ with oxygen inlet and non-return valve

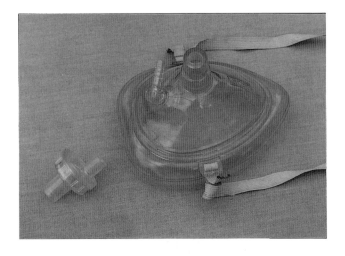

Some pocket-type masks are fitted with an oxygen inlet valve which can be attached, via oxygen supply tubing, to a constant flow oxygen system Laerdal claim that the Pocket Mask™ with an oxygen inlet may give inspired oxygen concentrations of up to 80% with a flow rate of 15 lpm, to a spontaneously breathing person. They can also be used for rescue breathing with oxygen supplementation, and Laerdal specify that with a flow rate of 10 lpm oxygen concentrations of up to 50% have been achieved in oxygen-assisted rescue breathing. Increasing the flow rate to 15 lpm can raise the oxygen concentration to around 54%.

It may be possible to further increase the oxygen concentration by connecting a length of respiratory tubing (preferably greater than about 12") to the port of the mask and blowing through the tubing; which acts as a reservoir.

It has been reported that, with flows of 15 lpm and higher, oxygen concentrations up to 100% can be obtained during artificial ventilation. This is achieved by the rescuer intermittently blocking the breathing port with his tongue or finger and opening it when the chest rises to permit exhalation. (Safar, 1988) However, this technique may require a much higher flow rate than 15 lpm and may be capable of overdistending the lungs and causing a pulmonary barotrauma. (Corry, 1990) *Consequently, DAN strongly recommends this technique never be attempted.*

Resuscitation masks, such as the Pocket Mask™, are capable of delivering larger tidal volumes than the bag-valve devices (described later), since both hands can be used to maintain airway patency and a secure mask fit. Up to 4 liters of reserve volume (i.e. the first aider's vital capacity) is available to compensate for leaks.

Some brands of pocket-style masks incorporate an inhalation/exhalation port with an outside diameter of 15 mm, enabling them to be attached to appropriate demand valves.

FIGURE 8.22

Ventilating a person using a Pocket Mask™

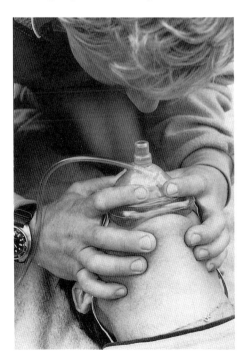

When using a pocket-style mask to provide oxygen to an adequately breathing diver:

- Ensure the injured diver is breathing adequately.
- Reassure a conscious diver, ask permission to provide oxygen and explain what you are doing.
- Position the diver appropriately. An unconscious diver should be placed in the recovery position.
- Ensure the area is well ventilated and that there is nothing burning in the immediate vicinity.
- Prepare the oxygen supply.
- Ensure the tubing is attached firmly to the nipple on the mask.
- Set the flow rate to 15 lpm. If the diver is suffering from decompression illness, it is better to give a high concentration as soon as possible and to continue until the supply is exhausted.
- If the diver is unconscious, place the mask over their nose and mouth with the narrow end over the nose. Position the supporting band around the diver's head and/or hold the mask firmly to their face, ensuring the best seal possible.
- Ask a conscious diver to place the mask over their mouth and nose with the narrow end upwards, and to hold it tightly to the face.
- Ask them to take deep, slow breaths.
- Record the periods of oxygen breathing and the diver's response.
- Carefully monitor the diver's condition by checking the airway, breathing, pulse and color.
- Carefully monitor the oxygen supply and remove the mask immediately if the supply becomes exhausted.
- Never leave the injured diver unattended.

When ventilating an inadequately breathing or non-breathing diver using a pocket-style mask:

- Position the diver flat on the back.
- Commence rescue breathing immediately and continue while the oxygen equipment is being prepared by another first aider. Check the carotid pulse. Feel for any resistance to inflation. If there is resistance, ensure the airway is adequately open and clear before continuing.
- Ensure the area is well ventilated and that there is nothing burning in the immediate vicinity.
- Prepare the oxygen supply.
- Ensure the oxygen tubing is attached firmly to the nipple on the mask.
- Mount the one-way valve on the mask port, if desired. Direct the exhalation valve away from you.
- Set the flow rate to 15 lpm.
- Place the mask over the diver's nose and mouth with the narrow end over the nose, ensuring the best seal possible.
- Tilt the diver's head back and lift the jaw. It is often convenient to position yourself behind the injured diver's head and open the airway using jaw thrust.
- Continue ventilating the diver at the appropriate rate.
- Monitor the diver's color and pulse and act accordingly. Commence external chest compressions, if required.
- Never leave the injured diver unattended.

Note:

If cross infection is a concern, fit the one-way valve and commence rescue breathing using the pocket-style mask immediately. When the oxygen supply is prepared, the oxygen tubing can be quickly attached to the mask and rescue breathing continued.

BAG-VALVE-MASK SYSTEMS

A bag-valve resuscitator can be used in conjunction with a tight-sealing mask or with advanced airways (e.g. endotracheal). A bag-valve-mask device consists of a self-inflating bag attached, via a mechanism with several one-way valves, to a tight-sealing mask. When the bag is compressed, air (and/or oxygen) is directed into the injured person by one-way valves. After compression, the bag automatically recoils and draws in air from the atmosphere (and/or oxygen from a reservoir). The injured person's exhaled breath is vented directly to the atmosphere and is prevented from entering the bag by a one-way valve.

There are a number of bag-valve-mask devices on the market. The manufacturers include Life Support Products, Laerdal and Ambu. These devices are designed for ventilating a non-breathing person in situations when direct contact is not desired. Since they deliver air, such systems provide an oxygen concentration of 21%, which is higher than the 16 to 17% in expired breath. However, most incorporate an oxygen inlet nipple so that supplemental oxygen can be given to increase the oxygen concentration. Some of these units are specified as being capable of providing up to 73% oxygen at a flow rate of 10 lpm, rising to almost 90% oxygen at a flow rate of 15 lpm (without using a reservoir bag). However, it is highly unlikely these concentrations would be achieved in the field.

The bags and masks come in sizes suitable for either adults, children or infants. Most newer models of adult bags have a volume of around 1600 ml. Older units often have bags with volumes of 1000-1200 ml. An adult system should not be used on a child since the bag is capable of overinflating the child's lungs. Some children's systems, as well as having smaller bags, incorporate an overpressure valve to prevent overinflation of the lungs.

Bag-valve-mask systems require extensive, specialized training to operate effectively and regular practice to maintain an adequate level of skill. They should only be used by those with appropriate training and skill. Such devices are not recommended by DAN for use by individuals without appropriate training and experience.

The current models of bag-valve-mask systems incorporate both an oxygen inlet and a plastic reservoir bag (or tube) which is usually attached to the tail of the self-inflating bag. Oxygen flows into both the resuscitator bag and the reservoir bag. When the resuscitator bag recoils, it initially draws in the contents of the reservoir and supplements it with air taken from the atmosphere until it has fully refilled.

As the oxygen flow rate is increased, more oxygen flows into the reservoir, which means that less air is drawn in to supplement the filling of the resuscitator bag.

For effective oxygenation during ventilations, the bag-valve device must have a supplemental oxygen inflow equal to or greater than the respiratory minute volume of the injured person. In addition, the reservoir bag should have a volume equal to or greater than the volume of the recoil bag. This should be greater than the injured person's tidal volume.

FIGURE 8.23
A Laerdal bag-valve-mask resuscitator

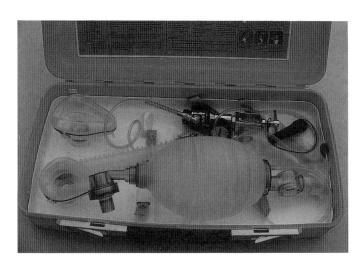

Units incorporating a reservoir are capable of providing oxygen concentrations of 95 to 100% at a flow rate of 10 to 15 lpm. However, when measured in actual practice, it is seldom greater than 95%. The oxygen concentration is reduced substantially if the seal is poor (which is common), or if the injured person is large and/or hyperventilating. (For example, with a good seal and a flow rate of 10 lpm, Laerdal specify that its bag-valve-mask system (with reservoir) can deliver an oxygen concentration of 100% to a person with a tidal volume of 750 ml and a breathing rate of 12 breaths per minute. However, with a person with a tidal volume of 1 liter and a breathing rate of 24 breaths per minute, it may deliver an oxygen concentration of only 53%.)

If near 100% oxygen is desired and the oxygen supply is limited, the best oxygen economy is obtained when flow is regulated so that the reservoir neither fills nor empties completely during ventilation cycles.

Bag-valve-mask systems can be used with conscious or unconscious, breathing persons; as well as with non-breathing persons. To ventilate a person, the oxygen provider has to first achieve an open airway and a good mask seal. It is often difficult to seal the mask onto the face and lift the jaw with one hand so the other hand is free to squeeze the bag. The injured person's mouth often closes under the mask and higher flows may be required to overcome nasal obstruction. The 1600 ml bag may not provide sufficient volume to compensate for leakage. However, if a good seal is achieved, bag-valve devices can provide sufficiently high pressures to inflate the stomach or damage the lungs. (Corry, 1990; Safar, 1988)

One interesting report describes an experiment during which 320 emergency medical technicians were required to ventilate a pre-calibrated recording resuscitation manikin using both a bag-valve-mask device and a Laerdal Pocket Mask™. The mean ventilatory volume with the bag-valve-mask device was 641 ml, which is well below the ideal mininum of 800 ml. More than 50% of the technicians were unable to ventilate the manikin to 800 ml using the bag-valve-mask device. In contrast, the mean ventilatory volume achieved using the Pocket Mask™ was 999 ml. (Elling, 1983)

Another series of experiments involved 35 hospital staff members who were required to ventilate a manikin to 800 ml. After instruction, their performance was satisfactory with mouth-to-mouth, mouth-to-mask and with a manually triggered oxygen-powered resuscitator (described later). However, bag-valve-mask resuscitation had a 97% failure rate. (Lawrence, 1985)

The leakage problems can be minimized by regular practice and various useful techniques, such as using your knees to help maintain head tilt. Extension tubes which allow the bag to be squeezed between the elbow and waist, so freeing up one hand, are available. If another first aider is available, they can be used to squeeze the bag so that the initial first aider can use two hands to obtain an adequate airway and seal. *Bag-valve-mask devices are used most effectively by at least two well-trained and experienced oxygen providers working together.* Indeed, because of the problems caused by ineffective use of such devices, some EMS systems now require that two rescuers operate bag-valve devices.

To optimize bag-valve-mask performance, one oxygen provider must be positioned at the top of the injured person's head. Generally an oropharyngeal airway (described later) should be inserted. The bag is squeezed slowly and the tidal volume is delivered over two seconds.

In addition to the problems previously described, in situations when a high concentration of oxygen is required (such as when treating decompression illness) most bag-valve-mask systems are not as economical on oxygen as are demand systems. For example, at a flow rate of 12 to 15 lpm, which is the flow rate required to provide high oxygen concentrations, a jumbo D cylinder would be exhausted in about 43 to 64 minutes. However, if a non-breathing person is being ventilated and the oxygen supply runs out, the oxygen provider can continue to ventilate the person since the resuscitator bag will still supply air (21% oxygen).

One available bag-valve device, manufactured by Life Support Products Inc., incorporates a bag-valve resuscitator as well as the Bag Refill-Valve described earlier. With this device, the resuscitator bag refills with 100% oxygen drawn from the Bag Refill-Valve. As a result, this system is more economical with oxygen than the other bag-valve devices, and 100% oxygen delivery can be achieved relatively easily. The LSP Bag Refill-Valve comes with adapters that fit other available bag-valve devices.

"An adequate bag-valve unit should have:

(1) a self-refilling bag that is easily cleaned and sterilized; (2) a nonjam valve system allowing for a minimum oxygen inlet flow of 15 lpm; (3) a no-pop-off valve; (4) standard 15 mm/22 mm fittings; (5) a system for delivering high concentrations of oxygen through an ancillary oxygen inlet at the back of the bag or via an oxygen reservoir; and (6) a true non-rebreathing valve. It should also (7) perform satisfactorily under all common environmental conditions and extremes of temperature; and (8) be available in adult and pediatric sizes." (JAMA, 1992)

FIGURE 8.24

Ventilating a person using the LSP bag-valve resuscitator and Bag Refill-Valve

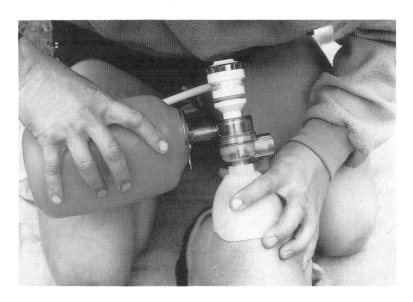

When using a constant flow bag-valve-mask system to provide oxygen to a breathing diver:

- Ensure the injured diver is breathing adequately.
- Reassure a conscious diver, ask permission to provide oxygen and explain what you are doing.
- Position the diver appropriately. An unconscious diver should be placed in the recovery position.
- Ensure the area is well ventilated and that there is nothing burning in the immediate vicinity.
- Prepare the oxygen supply.
- Ensure the oxygen tubing is attached firmly to the nipple on the bag-valve-mask device.
- Set the flow rate to 15 lpm. If the diver is suffering from decompression illness, it is better to give a high concentration as soon as possible and to continue until the supply is exhausted.
- Check that the oxygen is flowing through to the mask.
- If the diver is unconscious, place the mask over their nose and mouth with the narrow end over the nose and hold the mask firmly to their face, ensuring the best seal possible. Care must be taken not to obstruct the airway.
- Ask a conscious diver to place the mask over their mouth and nose with the narrow end upwards, and to hold it tightly to their face.
- Ask the diver to take deep, slow breaths.
- Record the periods of oxygen breathing and the diver's response.
- Carefully monitor the diver's condition by checking the airway, breathing, pulse and color.
- Carefully monitor the oxygen supply and remove the mask immediately if the supply becomes exhausted.
- Never leave the injured diver unattended.

WARNING:

It requires special skills to ventilate a person with a bag-valve-mask device. These skills can only be gained through appropriate training and adequate continuing practice. Such devices should never be used by those not trained to do so and are best used by two skilled operators.

When ventilating a diver using a constant flow bag-valve-mask system:

- Position the injured diver flat on the back.
- Commence rescue breathing immediately and continue while the oxygen equipment is being prepared by another oxygen provider. Check the carotid pulse.
- Ensure the area is well ventilated and that there is nothing burning in the immediate vicinity.
- Prepare the oxygen supply.
- Ensure the tubing is attached firmly to the nipple on the bag-valve-mask device.
- Set the flow rate to 15 lpm. If the diver is suffering from decompression illness, it is better to give a high oxygen concentration as soon as possible and to continue until the supply is exhausted.
- Check that the valves are functioning correctly by squeezing the bag.
- Place the mask over the diver's nose and mouth with the narrow end over the nose, ensuring the best seal possible.
- Position yourself behind the diver's head. Use one hand to open the airway using head tilt and jaw thrust while holding the mask to the injured diver's face.
- Use the other hand to ventilate the diver by squeezing the bag just enough to cause the lower chest and abdomen to rise. (If two first aiders are available one can maintain the airway and mask seal while the other squeezes the bag.) *Stop squeezing as soon as the chest rises.*
- Feel for any resistance to inflation. If there is resistance, ensure the airway adequately open and clear before continuing.
- Continue to ventilate the diver at the appropriate rate.
- Monitor the diver's color and pulse and act accordingly.
- Never leave the injured diver unattended.

Note: If you are unable to ventilate the diver effectively using the bag-valve-mask device, abandon the device and revert to rescue breathing without delay.

CLOSED CIRCUIT OXYGEN RESUSCITATION DEVICES

In most oxygen units the injured person's exhaled gas is exhausted into the atmosphere. If a person is breathing near 100% oxygen, only 4 to 5% of their expired breath is carbon dioxide and most of the balance is oxygen. It seems wasteful not to use this expired oxygen.

Various closed circuit oxygen "rebreathing" devices have been produced. These units are capable of delivering very high oxygen concentrations while extending the duration of the oxygen cylinder very substantially. The duration of a cylinder which may normally last around 40 minutes can sometimes be extended to 6 hours or longer. This provides obvious advantages if oxygen needs to be provided for a prolonged period and the oxygen supply is limited. The main benefit is to divers who dive in very remote locations.

Most units incorporate a cannister of soda lime, a chemical which absorbs carbon dioxide. Instead of being exhaled to the atmosphere, the injured person's exhaled gas flows through the soda lime where carbon dioxide is removed. The remaining gas, which is mainly oxygen and water vapor, remains in the system, where, after being supplemented with extra oxygen, it is rebreathed. This process can continue until the inflowing fresh oxygen supply is depleted.

As with any oxygen system, the inspired oxygen concentration depends largely on the effectiveness of the seal. However, an additional problem may arise with a closed circuit system when used to treat a sufferer of decompression illness.

Excess nitrogen remains in our body for many hours after a dive. When treating decompression illness, it is important to try to completely exclude nitrogen from the breathing gas in order to maximize the washout of nitrogen from the diver's body.

In a closed circuit oxygen system, some of the excess nitrogen exhaled by the diver may be trapped in the system. Although, after normal recreational diving activities this volume of nitrogen would not be very large, these systems should be flushed periodically to remove accumulated nitrogen. However, at present, there appears to be no available data on how often the system needs to be flushed to eliminate nitrogen. Recommended flushing procedures are provided with some units. One general procedure that has been suggested is to flush the system after 5 minutes, after a further 15 minutes, and every 15 to 30 minutes thereafter. This procedure has been shown to be effective in maintaining near 100% oxygen concentrations in normobaric studies of nitrogen elimination.

A closed circuit system must also be flushed appropriately if used to provide oxygen to a person who is suffering from toxic gas inhalation.

There are several other potential problems with closed circuit devices:

The soda lime needs to be changed regularly. Users must be familiar with the particular granules used in the system so that they know when the granules need to be replaced. Active granules will become warm when the system is being used, but this does not imply exhaustion of the soda lime. Usually there is a depletion indicator which changes color (often from white to purple) when the soda lime is exhausted. **If the granules are exhausted and the unit is used, carbon dioxide will be recirculated and the injured diver could suffer from severe carbon dioxide toxicty. Consequently, it is essential to ensure the soda lime granules are active and to monitor the diver carefully.**

It has been reported that, if soda lime is not packed correctly, soda lime dust may be inhaled and may cause complications. However, this appears to be rare. In additon, if soda lime crystals get very wet (not just damp), as they could on a dive boat unless the unit is adequately sealed, they will not remove the carbon dioxide effectively.

Finally, most portable closed circuit devices utilize a soft bag that relies on an oxygen supply and an excellent seal in order to reinflate. A skilled operator can easily monitor the injured person's breathing and determine whether the airway is obstructed, and, with some devices, can resuscitate a non-breathing person. However, it can be extremely difficult for an operator who is not highly skilled to ventilate an injured diver effectively.

Closed circuit devices should not be used by those without adequate training and practice.

FIGURE 8.25

Wenoll closed circuit oxygen system

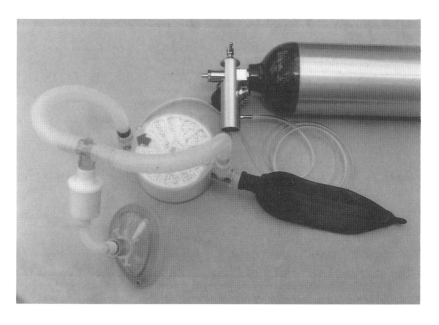

REVIEW QUESTIONS

1. List some benefits of clear resuscitation masks.

2. What is the easiest and most effective system for delivering 100% oxygen to a breathing diver?

3. How may a poor mask seal affect the functioning of a demand valve?

4. How can a demand system which is not fitted with a ventilation button be used to provide a high oxygen concentration to a non-breathing diver?

5. Why are constant flow delivery devices usually uneconomical on oxygen?

6. On what factors does the oxygen concentration delivered by a constant flow system depend?

7. Why does it require extensive training and practice to use a bag-valve-mask device to provide resuscitation?

8. What are the potential hazards of using a manually triggered oxygen-powered device for resuscitation?

9. What are the potential problems of using a closed circuit oxygen device?

TABLE 8.2

Potential oxygen concentrations and applications of various delivery devices

Delivery device	% O$_2$	Condition of casualty		
		Cons.	Uncons. Breath.	Non-breath.
LSP demand inhalator valve	100	Y	Y	N
LSP Bag Refill-Valve	100	Y	Y	N
LSP CPR/demand valve	100	Y	Y	Y
Elder CPR/demand valve	100	Y	Y	Y
MTV	100	Y	Y	Y
Nasal cannula	24- 44 at 1-6 lpm	Y	Y	with RB
Simple face mask	35-60 at 6-14 lpm	Y	Y	N
Partial rebreather mask	60 at 10 lpm	Y	Y	N
Non rebreather mask	95 at 10 -15 lpm	Y	Y	N
Pocket Mask™	54-80 at 15 lpm	Y	Y	with RB
Bag valve-mask device (with reservoir)	95-100 at 10 -15 lpm	Y	Y	Y

Note: It is emphasized that the oxygen concentrations achievable using different delivery devices vary from one report to another. The concentrations quoted here are usually the maximum possible. The oxygen concentration actually achieved when some of this equipment is used in the field, and/or by an operator who is unfamiliar with it, is likely to be substantially lower than that quoted.

Chapter 9

THE DAN OXYGEN UNIT

As previously mentioned, although there are a variety of oxygen systems available, much of it is unsuitable for the general diving public. To remedy this situation, the Divers Alert Network assembled an oxygen unit designed specifically to cater to divers' requirements. DAN currently endorses this specific system for divers who are medical laypersons.

The DAN Oxygen Unit is not only effective, but also easy to use and requires minimal training. DAN has developed a four hour training program designed to develop skills and confidence assembling and operating the DAN Oxygen Unit and to help participants understand the effects of working with oxygen. CPR certification is required prior to entering the course. A training video is also available to refresh skills and knowledge.

The DAN Oxygen Unit contains an LSP multi-function regulator, demand inhalator valve with clear Tru-Fit™ mask, Laerdal Pocket Mask™, non-rebreather mask with six-foot oxygen tubing, jumbo D cylinder, valve-wrench/hand wheel with chain, and waterproof King Pelican case. The complete unit is available directly from DAN.

FIGURE 9.1
DAN Oxygen Unit

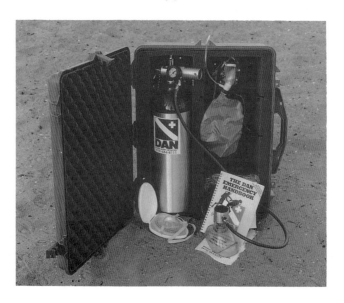

DAN also distribute a "Mini" DAN Oxygen Unit. The Mini Unit has all the component parts found in the standard unit, except that it has no cylinder and is housed in a smaller (# 1400) Pelican case.

The demand valve can be used to supply 100% oxygen to a breathing diver, whether conscious or unconscious. A second injured diver can be treated with a high oxygen concentration by using the non-rebreather mask attached to the barbed constant flow outlet. In the event that a breathing diver cannot tolerate the demand inhalator valve, or if there is a second breathing injured diver, the regulator constant flow feature can be used with a non-rebreather mask. If an injured diver needs to be ventilated, this can be achieved in a relatively safe and effective manner by using the Pocket Mask™ attached, via oxygen tubing, to the barbed outlet.

THE COMPONENTS OF THE DAN OXYGEN UNIT

Multi-function Regulator

The regulator, manufactured by Life Support Products Inc., is a one piece pressure reducer for use with oxygen. It is a multi-function piston regulator with two high pressure DISS threaded outlet ports (each with check valves) which flow at rates exceeding 100 lpm at a pressure of 40 to 60 psi. In addition, there is one barbed outlet with a flow selector knob that provides flow rate settings of 1, 2, 4, 6, 10, 15 and 25 lpm. It also incorporates a sturdy pressure gauge, protected by a rubber boot. The regulator is pictured in Figure 7.6

The regulator, which is made from anodized aluminum, is durable and can be used in temperatures ranging from -30°F to 125°F. It is designed for use with oxygen cylinders with pressures ranging from 2200 psi down to 500 psi. It incorporates a pressure relief valve to protect the injured person and the delivery devices in the event of first stage failure. The relief valve is set to blow off at about 85 psi. Although the standard DAN unit is fitted with a pin-indexed yoke, a CGA-540 threaded fitting is also available for use with larger (H and M) oxygen cylinders.

LSP demand inhalator valve

The demand valve used in the DAN Oxygen Unit is an LSP demand inhalator valve (Figure 8.3), specifically designed without a positive pressure activating button. The body of the valve is made from anodized aluminum. LSP Inc. specifies that it takes 0 to -2 cm H_2O to crack the valve and start the flow of oxygen, which will flow to 160 lpm or to the maximum flow capacity of the regulator, which in this unit is over 100 lpm. There is little or no resistance caused by the valve. The specified exhalation resistance is from 1.5 to 6.4 cm H_2O, depending on the flow rate.

Laerdal Pocket Mask™

The Laerdal Pocket Mask™ is fitted with an oxygen inlet valve which can be attached, via oxygen tubing, to the barbed constant flow outlet on the regulator. When used for rescue breathing with oxygen supplementation with a flow rate of 15 lpm, oxygen concentrations of 54% have been achieved with a Pocket

Mask™. In addition, such masks may provide oxygen concentrations of up to 80% to a breathing person, when used with a flow rate of 15 lpm. DAN recommends a minimum flow rate of 15 lpm.

The Pocket Mask™ is a resuscitation adjunct that is a reasonable substitute for manually triggered oxygen-powered or bag-valve-mask positive pressure ventilations since it requires far less training and continued practice than the other devices. Resuscitation masks, such as the Laerdal Pocket Mask™, are capable of delivering larger tidal volumes than the bag-valve devices, since both hands can be used to maintain airway patency and a secure mask fit.

The Pocket Mask™ can be used on the demand inhalator valve in place of the Tru Fit™ mask for those injured divers with small faces, beards or other unusual facial features.

Non-rebreather mask

This mask, described in Chapter 8, is fitted with a 750 ml reservoir bag which fills with oxygen. When the injured diver inhales, a one-way valve ensures the diver breathes primarily oxygen from the reservoir.

For proper use, the reservoir bag must be primed before it is fitted to the diver and should always contain enough oxygen so that it does not deflate fully. In addition, all three one-way valves should be fitted and seating properly and a good seal needs to be achieved. Under optimal conditions, non-rebreather masks have been reported to deliver oxygen concentrations up to 95% at flow rates of 10 to 15 lpm. DAN recommends a minimum flow rate of 15 lpm when using such a device. The flow rate should be increased, if necessary, to prevent the reservoir bag from deflating completely.

Although a non-rebreather mask is not capable of supplying as high oxygen concentrations as the demand inhalator valve with tight-sealing mask, it can be very useful if an injured diver has difficulty with the demand system, or if there are two injured divers requiring oxygen.

Oxygen tubing

Six feet of oxygen tubing is supplied. The tubing is actually part of the non-rebreather mask which is supplied with the unit. It can be removed from the mask and attached to the Laerdal Pocket Mask™, if necessary. One end of the tubing should be attached to the barbed constant flow outlet and the other end to the non-rebreather mask or Laerdal Pocket Mask™.

Case

The unit comes in a "King" Pelican case, which is sturdy, waterproof and buoyant, and which contains additional storage.

Cylinder

The cylinder is an aluminum Jumbo D cylinder which contains approximately 636 liters of oxygen.

USING THE DAN OXYGEN UNIT

To prepare the oxygen supply:

- Ensure the area is well ventilated and that there is nothing burning in the immediate vicinity (including cigarettes).
- Ensure that the cylinder valve and regulator fitting are clean and free from any oil or grease.
- Remove the oxygen unit from the case, as necessary, and lay the unit beside the injured diver, keeping the cylinder away from their head.
- Grasp the shoulder of the cylinder with the pressure gauge pointed away from youself and others.
- Attach the wrench to the cylinder if necessary.
- Set the constant flow dial to zero.
- Slowly open the cylinder valve counter-clockwise and pressurize the regulator.
- Turn off the valve and observe the pressure gauge to detect leaks.
- Rectify any leaks (check sealing washer).
- Open the cylinder valve one full turn.
- Check the pressure gauge to determine how much oxygen is available. If system fails to pressurize, the cylinder is empty and cannot be used.

Conscious diver

To maximize the inhaled oxygen concentration, the demand inhalator valve attached to the Tru-Fit™ mask or Pocket Mask™ should be used.

However, if a spontaneously breathing diver cannot breathe effectively through the demand inhalator valve, the non-rebreather mask can be used instead. The non-rebreather mask can also be use to treat a second injured (breathing) diver when the demand inhalator valve is already being used.

When using the demand inhalator valve with a conscious diver:

- Reassure a conscious diver, ask permission to provide oxygen and explain what you are doing.
- Position the injured diver appropriately. If decompression illness is suspected, the diver should be laid down flat. Heart attack sufferers or asthmatics may prefer to be semi-reclined or sitting upright as they are often less breathless in this position.
- Attach the the Tru-Fit™ mask or Pocket Mask™ to the demand inhalator valve and breathe from the demand valve to ensure that it is performing adequately.
- Position the mask carefully over the diver's nose and mouth with the narrow end over the nose and the chin cup (if using the Tru Fit™) under the chin. Ensure the best seal possible. Encouraging the diver to hold the mask themself may provide some reassurance.
- Ask the injured diver to breathe slowly and deeply.
- Record the periods of oxygen breathing and the diver's response.
- Carefully monitor the oxygen supply and remove the mask immediately if the supply becomes exhausted, or the diver cannot breathe from the demand valve.
- Carefully monitor the injured diver's condition and never leave them unattended.

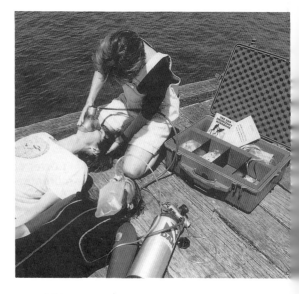

FIGURE 9.2

Two conscious divers breathing oxygen from the DAN Unit.

Unconscious spontaneously breathing diver

Once again, the demand inhalator valve attached to the Tru-Fit™ mask or Pocket Mask™ should be used, if possible, to maximize the inspired oxygen concentration. The unconscious diver must be monitored very carefully and the oxygen provider must ensure the demand inhalator valve is being triggered effectively by the injured diver's breathing.

If there is difficulty with using the demand inhalator valve, the non-rebreather mask can be used as a reasonable alternative.

When using the demand inhalator valve with an unconscious, breathing diver:

- Place the injured diver in the recovery position, ensure the airway is clear and open the airway by head tilt and chin lift or jaw thrust.
- Attach the Tru-Fit™ mask or Pocket Mask™ to the demand inhalator valve and breathe from the demand valve to ensure that it is performing adequately.
- Position the mask carefully over the diver's nose and mouth with the narrow end over the nose. Ensure the best seal possible or the demand valve may not function effectively.
- Record the periods of oxygen breathing and the diver's response.
- Carefully monitor the injured diver's condition by checking the airway, breathing, pulse and color.
- Carefully monitor the oxygen supply and remove the mask immediately if the supply becomes exhausted.
- Never leave the injured diver unattended.

When using the non-rebreather mask:

- Ensure the injured diver is breathing adequately.
- Reassure a conscious diver, ask permission to provide oxygen and explain what you are doing.
- Position the diver appropriately. An unconscious, breathing diver should be placed in the recovery position.
- Prepare the oxygen supply and set the flow rate to 15 lpm. DAN recommends a minimum flow rate of 15 lpm for diving accidents.
- Cover the valve by placing your thumb inside the nosepiece to allow the reservoir bag to fully inflate.
- Ask a conscious diver to place the mask over their mouth and nose with the narrow end upwards and the metal band (if fitted) over the bridge of the nose.
- Ask the diver to take deep, slow breaths.
- Explain what you are doing and that the hissing sound is oxygen flowing into the mask.
- Position the supporting band around the diver's head and tighten until secure. The fit can be improved (and eye irritation minimized) by gently squeezing the metal band so that it fits snugly onto the nose.
- Record the periods of oxygen breathing and the diver's response.
- Carefully monitor the injured diver's condition by checking the airway, breathing, pulse and color and act accordingly.
- Carefully monitor the oxygen supply and remove the mask immediately if the supply becomes exhausted.
- Never leave the injured diver unattended.

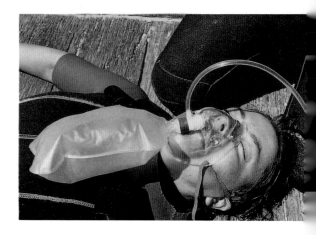

FIGURE 9.3

Using a non-rebreather mask

Unconscious non-breathing diver

To ventilate a non-breathing diver with the DAN Oxygen Unit, an oxygen provider can perform oxygen-supplemented rescue breathing via the Laerdal Pocket Mask™.

When ventilating a diver using the Pocket Mask™:

- Position the injured diver flat on the back.
- Commence rescue breathing immediately and continue while the oxygen equipment is being prepared by another oxygen provider.
- Ensure the tubing is attached firmly to the oxygen nipple on the Pocket Mask™.
- Mount the one-way valve on the mask port. Direct the exhalation valve away from you.
- Set the flow rate to 15 lpm.
- Place the mask over the diver's nose and mouth with the narrow end over the nose, ensuring the best seal possible.
- Tilt the injured diver's head back and lift the jaw.
- Continue ventilating the diver at the appropriate rate.
- Monitor the diver's color and pulse and act accordingly.
- Never leave the injured diver unattended.

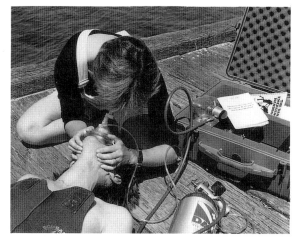

FIGURE 9.4

Ventilating a non-breathing diver using a Pocket Mask™

REVIEW QUESTIONS

1. How may the DAN Oxygen Unit be used to provide near 100% oxygen to an injured diver who is breathing spontaneously?

2. If an injured diver who is breathing spontaneously has difficulty breathing from the demand inhalator valve of the DAN Oxygen Unit, what other piece of equipment should be used to maximize the oxygen concentration delivered ?

3. What flow rate should be selected when using the non-rebreather mask?

4. How can the DAN Oxygen Unit be used to provide elevated oxygen concentrations when resuscitating a non-breathing diver?

Chapter 10

ADJUNCTIVE EQUIPMENT FOR AIRWAY MANAGEMENT

10.1 SUCTION DEVICES

Suction can be very effective in aspirating fluid matter such as mucus, saliva and vomit from the mouth and nose of an unconscious person to prevent inhalation of the fluids and help clear the airway. Fluids are removed prior to oxygen resuscitation since, as in all resuscitation procedures, a clear airway is absolutely essential. Suction can also be used during resuscitation if there is a further accumulation of fluids in the mouth. However, suction cannot remove solid matter and some viscous mucus, which should be removed with the fingers.

Many oxygen resuscitation units are provided with suction and independent suction devices are also available. Some suction is powered by oxygen. In such units, a rapid flow of oxygen is directed past an opening on or near the collection bottle. This has a venturi effect and creates a vacuum in the bottle, thereby providing the suction. *Oxygen-powered suction should be used sparingly as it rapidly uses the oxygen supply.* However, suction is rarely required for longer than 15-20 seconds. The valve should be turned off immediately after use. Other units are powered by air, batteries, hand, foot and various other sources.

FIGURE 10.1.1

LSP oxygen-powered suction device

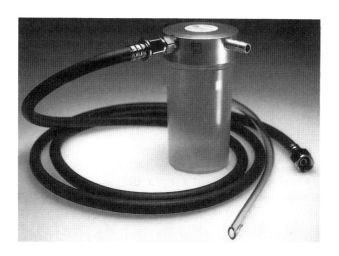

FIGURE 10.1.2

Laerdal battery-powered (left) and Vivac hand-powered (right) suction devices

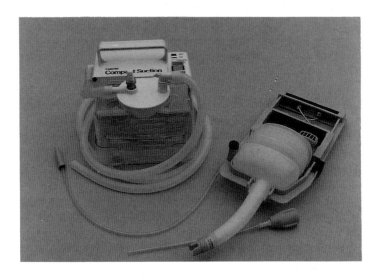

Suction devices should include a vacuum source, a control valve, a nonbreakable collection bottle, a large-bore, non-kinking connecting tube, sterile semi-rigid suction tips and sterile catheters of various sizes. Most suction catheters and tips have a finger port (air vent) that can be sealed and unsealed by the first aider's finger to control suction. Ideally, such a device should provide a negative pressure of at least 400 cmH2O when the tube is occluded, and a minimum air flow of 30 lpm when the tube is open. The amount of suction should be controllable for use on small persons. The suction control, collection bottle, sterile water for rinsing and suction tube should be readily accessible to the first aider in charge of the airway. The tube should reach the airway of the injured diver regardless of their position. Suction devices must be designed for easy cleaning and decontamination.

In the absence of a suspected spinal injury, when suction is used the injured diver is often best positioned either with the head turned to the side or in the recovery posion. This enables fluids to drain to the lower cheek.

The first aider holds the suction catheter like a pencil and inserts it into the diver's mouth *taking care never to place it further in than the back teeth (ea. lobe).* **If the injured diver is not deeply unconscious, placing a suction catheter into the throat further than the back teeth may cause gagging or vomiting and the associated complications.**

Suction is not applied while the catheter is being inserted. The catheter is carefully placed to its proper depth and suction is applied while it is being withdrawn. The catheter is gently swept across the lower cheek. It should not be left still for more than a few seconds since it can dry up and block on mucous membrane. The line should be flushed periodically with water to keep the sucker patent. This can be achieved by inserting the catheter into a bowl of water and aspirating the water to clear the catheter and tubing.

Suction must be timed so as not to interfere with the diver's spontaneous breathing or with controlled ventilation.

To test the suction, place a finger or thumb over the end of the tubing (without the catheter attached) and turn on the suction. There should be enough suction to hold the tube to the finger or thumb. If the suction is not working effectively, check: (1) there is an oxygen supply and it is turned on (oxygen-powered units only); (2) that the lid of the collection bottle is tight; (3) the seal inside the lid of the bottle is in place and in good condition; and (4) there are no cracks in the bottle or kinks or cracks in the tubing.

When using suction:

- Position the injured diver appropriately.
- Clear solid matter from the airway with finger sweeps.
- Tilt the head and support the jaw, as appropriate.
- Select and fit the appropriate suction catheter.
- Turn on the oxygen if the suction is oxygen-powered.
- Turn on the suction and check that it is working.
- Open the unconscious diver's mouth.
- Carefully and gently insert the catheter to the appropriate depth *taking care not to place it beyond the back teeth.*
- Aspirate the diver by occluding the catheter control hole, if present.
- Sweep the catheter across the lower cheek while withdrawing the catheter.
- Avoid aspirating for more than 5 seconds at a time.
- Flush the line with water.
- Ensure the suction bottle does not fill beyond two-thirds full. Empty it if necessary.

Note:

If an oropharyngeal airway is in place, carry out the above procedure, aspirating inside and on both sides of the oropharyngeal airway. If suctioning the nostrils, suction each nostril separately while closing the other nostril.

10.2 OROPHARYNGEAL AIRWAYS

WARNING: Special training and frequent practice are required prior to inserting an oropharyngeal airway. Such devices must only be used by specially trained personnel, and only on an unconscious person who does not display a gag reflex.

Oropharyngeal airways are sometimes used to maintain a patent airway. Correctly inserted, they prevent airway obstruction by the tongue, lips and teeth.

It may be necessary to insert an oropharyngeal airway to avoid generating excessive airway pressures when using devices such as a manually triggered oxygen-powered resuscitator with mask, a bag-valve-mask device or a pocket-style mask to ventilate a non-breathing diver.

Oropharyngeal airways are made from a firm plastic or rubber. They are curved to follow the shape of the pharynx and come in a variety of sizes to suit different sizes of injured persons - large adult, adult, child, infant, newborn and others. There are at least seven sizes available. It is important to use only the correct size. The appropriate size airway is selected by placing it on the diver's face so that it measures from the center of the lip to the angle of the lower jaw as shown in Figure 10.2.2. Alternatively, with the airway reversed to follow the contour of the jaw, it can be measured from the corner of the injured diver's mouth, to the tip of the ear lobe on the same side of the face.

FIGURE 10.2.1

Various sizes of oropharyngeal airways

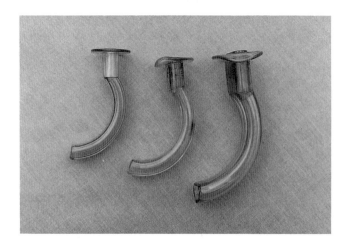

FIGURE 10.2.2

Measuring an oropharyngeal airway

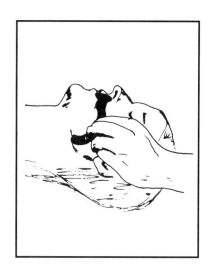

Oropharyngeal airways must only be used on an unconscious diver who does not display a gag reflex. If inserted in a conscious person whose upper airway gag reflexes are intact, an oropharyngeal airway can cause vomiting, laryngospasm and/or dental damage.

If an oropharyngeal airway is incorrectly inserted, the tongue may be pushed back into the pharynx and may obstruct the airway. Therefore, great care is needed when inserting such an airway. As previously mentioned, *special training and frequent practice are required prior to inserting an oropharyngeal airway. Such devices must only be used by trained personnel.*

INSERTION OF AN OROPHARYNGEAL AIRWAY

FIGURE 10.2.3

Inserting an oropharyngeal airway

Diagrams reproduced courtesy of Dr. D. Komesaroff

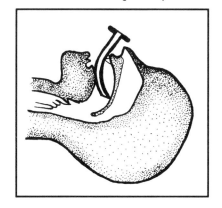 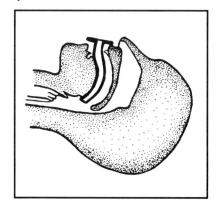

When inserting an oropharyngeal airway:

- Ensure the diver is unconscious and that the mouth is moderately relaxed.
- Clear the airway.
- Select the appropriate size oropharyngeal airway.
- If lubrication is necessary, lubricate the airway with water, a medical lubricant (e.g. KY jelly) or the injured diver's saliva (which may not be desirable if cross infection is a concern).
- Open the injured diver's mouth and apply head tilt and/or jaw thrust.
- Hold the airway by the flange with the natural curve upside down and the tip pointing towards the roof of the diver's mouth.
- Insert it tip first until about one-third of its length is into the mouth, above the tongue. Take care not to push the tongue back into the throat.
- Rotate the airway over the tongue so that it now points towards the side of the injured diver's mouth.
- Gently push the airway approximately two-thirds of its length into the diver's mouth, above the tongue, whilst continuing to rotate it so that the tip is pointing down the pharynx (i.e. it has been rotated a full 180°).
- Continue to gently insert it until the flange rests against the diver's lips, and the bite block is between the teeth.
- Do not continue to insert the airway if the diver opposes its insertion. Remove the airway immediately if the diver begins to cough, gag or vomit, or attempts to remove it with the tongue.
- Ensure the lower lip is not pinched between the teeth and the oral airway.
- Maintain head tilt and jaw support.
- Look, listen and feel for air movement.

REVIEW QUESTIONS

1. Why can suction be useful on an unconscious diver?
2. How far into the throat is a suction catheter inserted, and why no further?
3. Why is the catheter moved continuously when aspirating?
4. What equipment checks should be made if the suction is not working effectively?
5. Who may insert an oropharyngeal airway?
6. Why are oropharyngeal airways used?
7. Why must the diver be unconscious when an oropharyngeal airway is inserted

Chapter 11

CARE AND MAINTENANCE OF OXYGEN EQUIPMENT

When using oxygen equipment it is desirable to avoid allowing the cylinder to empty beyond the safe residual. However, if a cylinder is emptied, the valve should be turned off immediately to prevent moisture and other contaminants from entering.

The oxygen outlet should never be sealed with adhesive tape since most are petroleum based. A static electric spark can be generated when such tape is removed and, if oxygen has accumulated in the area, a fire could result. Never use grease, oil or fat-based soaps on any oxygen equipment.

It is important to pack and store oxygen equipment properly after use. The cylinder pressure should be read before turning off the valve. If the pressure is below about 1,500 psi the cylinder should be replaced and refilled. (This may not always be applicable to larger cylinders). The cylinder valve must never be left on in case oxygen escapes while the unit is stored. *The system should be depressurized and all flow valves turned off.* Depressurizing the system relieves the pressure on valve seats and lines and increases their lifetime. Masks, tubing and other parts requiring cleaning should be checked for wear, cleaned, disinfected and dried before being packed. Disposable items such as suction catheters should be thrown away after use and replaced with new ones.

Any missing items should be noted and replaced. Tubing should be carefully coiled to prevent kinking. Soft masks have a tendency to distort if squashed during storage. Such masks can be stuffed with tissue paper to help prevent distortion. All components should be checked carefully, reassembled if necessary and packed so that they can be quickly unpacked when required.

The unit should be stored in a secure and stable location to prevent it being tampered with and/or falling over. The location should be well ventilated and away from heat sources and combustible materials.

REVIEW QUESTIONS

1. Why is it desirable not to deplete an oxygen cylinder?
2. Why is the cylinder valve turned off and the system depressurized prior to storage?
3. Why is it important to ensure all components are present, functioning and packed correctly?
4. Why should the unit be stored away from heat sources and in a well ventilated area?

To ensure oxygen equipment is maintained and stored appropriately:

- Always ensure that the cylinder is full, and turned off, before storing.
- Depressurize the regulator before storing.
- Keep oxygen equipment clean, dry and in a safe location. Never allow oil, grease or other flammable substances to come into contact with the equipment.
- Store in a well ventilated area, away from sources of heat and combustible materials.
- Check the contents of the cylinder and functioning of the equipment regularly.
- Oxygen units should be inspected and serviced by an appropriately trained technician at regular intervals as specified by the manufacturer.
- Only refill the cylinder at authorized and reputable dealers.
- Cylinders must be visually and hydrostatically tested every 5-10 years, as specified. Ensure the cylinder is currently in test. If necessary, check with your gas supplier.
- Thoroughly wash, disinfect and dry the mask and other appropriate parts after use (See Chapter 12).
- Masks with an inflatable/inflated cuff should be replaced at the first sign of deterioration of the cuff.
- Spare sealing washers should be kept with the equipment.
- Most cases may be cleaned with soap (non fat-based) and water. However, plastic cases should not be cleaned with substances that adversely affect plastic.
- Consult the manufacturers' literature for more specific maintenance instructions.

Chapter 12

RISK OF CROSS INFECTION WHEN PROVIDING FIRST AID

There is a risk that some infections may be transmitted in the course of life saving activities. Certain blood-borne viruses such as Hepatitis B, Hepatitis C and the Human Immuno Deficiency Virus (HIV) have caused the greatest concern and will be the subject of this discussion. However, other infections such as Tuberculosis, Herpes Simplex (cold sores), colds, gastro-intestinal bacteria and upper respiratory infections may also be transmitted.

Since the dose of infected material required to transmit Hepatitis B is much lower than that required to transmit HIV, the risk of acquiring Hepatitis B is higher.

Although several body fluids can contain these viruses, blood and saliva are the most significant body fluids for emergency care providers to be concerned about. The risk of acquiring infection as a result of rescue or emergency care is directly proportional to the frequency of exposure to blood or saliva. Rescuers who are frequently exposed to blood have a greater chance of coming into contact with infected blood.

Vaccination against Hepatitis B has been shown to be effective and should be considered by those who are routinely exposed to risk of infection. However, currently there is no immunization for Hepatitis C or HIV, so care should be taken to avoid or minimize exposure, especially to blood. Where possible, a barrier such as disposable rubber gloves should be used to prevent direct contact with blood.

Saliva is normally considered to carry a relatively low risk of cross infection. However, transmission via saliva may become more of a problem if bleeding in the mouth occurs. Even in the absence of blood, the possibility of cross infection as a result of giving rescue breathing or when using a manikin for training purposes is currently causing concern.

"The probability that a rescuer (lay or professional) will become infected with Hepatitis B or HIV as a result of performing CPR is minimal. Although transmission of Hepatitis B or HIV between health care workers and patients has been documented as a result of blood exchange or penetration of the skin by blood-contaminated instruments, transmission of Hepatitis B or HIV during mouth-to-mouth resuscitation has not been documented." (JAMA, 1992)

Even though the risk of cross infection appears minimal, where possible a protective device such as a mask or face shield should be used. Rescuers who have a duty to provide CPR have been advised to use barriers, such as latex gloves, and mechanical ventilation equipment, such as a bag-valve-mask and other resuscitation masks with valves capable of diverting expired air from the rescuer. (MMWR, 1989) Masks without one-way valves (including those with S-shaped devices) offer little, if any, protection and should not be considered for routine use. (JAMA, 1992) However, the efficacy of such barrier devices may vary and new problems may be introduced. At the present time, there appears to be no conclusive evidence to show that the masks with additional one-way valves provide extra protection against cross infection. In addition, the one-way valves can occassionally malfunction. Face shields with filtered openings are also available. Although, their effectiveness in preventing disease transmission is yet to be proven, these may provide a degree of protection. Some face shields with filters can be very difficult to blow through when they become wet. However, it is important that the lack of proven efficacy and potential problems of certain barrier devices should not deter the first aider from using a barrier device; but should be considered when choosing which device(s) to include in a first aid kit.

In addition to the precautionary methods used while administering first aid, there are several measures to be taken afterwards. These include personal hygiene and the cleaning of equipment.

First aiders should wash their hands thoroughly with soap and water after administering first aid (or after using training manikins and rescuscitation equipment). Soap should be included in the first aid kit.

FIGURE 12.1

Various types of one-way valves and face shields

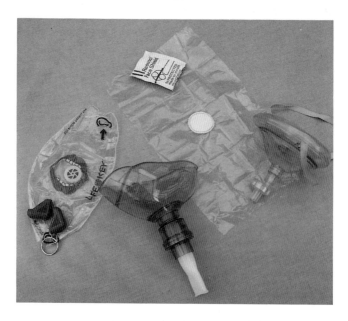

Manikins are used during resuscitation training. Studies have shown that it is theoretically possible to transfer organisms while using resuscitation training manikins in the absence of thorough disinfecting routines. A similar theoretical risk may apply to resuscitation equipment. Therefore, it is strongly recommended that manikins and resuscitation equipment be cleaned thoroughly and in accordance with the manufacturer's instructions. "Airway isolation" designed manikins are available and are preferable. Despite these concerns, at present there appears to be no documented evidence of transmission of bacterial, fungal, or viral disease through the use of resuscitation training manikins. (JAMA, 1992)

CLEANING RESUSCITATION EQUIPMENT

Resuscitation equipment must be thoroughly cleaned as soon as possible after use to prevent cross infection. Dried body substances are often more difficult to remove.

The equipment must then be brush-cleaned, disinfected, rinsed and dried prior to storage. Drying should prevent the survival and growth of fungal or bacterial pathogens while the equipment is stored. Prior to storage, the equipment should be checked for signs of deterioration. Cracks or tears in surfaces may make thorough cleaning impossible. Damaged parts should be replaced.

Specific cleaning instructions should be provided with the equipment, including a list of chemicals which are effective and compatible with the particular piece of equipment. These instructions should be carefully followed. Using inappropriate chemicals may fail to disinfect, cause certain parts to perish prematurely, cause adverse skin reactions or have an unpleasant taste or odor.

Some general rules for cleaning equipment are:

- Discard any disposable parts.
- Disassemble the equipment as appropriate.
- Pre-rinse the appropriate parts with cold, running water.
- Wash appropriate parts thoroughly in warm water using a detergent that is compatible with the resuscitator materials. Careful scrubbing with a soft brush can be effective.
- Rinse the parts thoroughly in clean, fresh water.
- Immerse the parts in the recommended sterilizing solution for the time specified.
- Rinse the parts thoroughly in clean, fresh water.
- Dry all parts thoroughly.
- Reassemble the equipment.
- Test the equipment after reassembly to ensure it operates correctly.

Sodium hypochlorite (500 parts per million of freshly made solution) is considered an appropriate broad spectrum disinfectant for *clean* surfaces. A suitable solution can be made by mixing 1/4 cup (60 ml) of liquid household bleach per 3.8 liters (one U.S. gallon) of tap water. Ten minute submersion has been suggested. The surface should be thoroughly precleaned to remove organic (and other) material since hypochlorite is substantially inactivated in the presence of blood. The solution must be freshly made, which means prepared within 24 hours of use.

REVIEW QUESTIONS

1. Which is the most significant body fluid for emergency care providers to be concerned about?

2. What aids can a rescuer use to minimize direct contact with blood?

3. How soon after use should resuscitation equipment be cleaned?

4. How is equipment precleaned prior to sterilization?

5. What should be done after the equipment has been sterilized?

Chapter 13

LEGAL CONSIDERATIONS

t common law there is no obligation to act as a "good samaritan" and an dividual is under no duty to rescue or provide first aid to a dying stranger. owever, having initiated first aid management, the rescuer is required to act in ccordance with training and experience, if any. Good Samaritan laws exist hroughout the United States. Laypersons are protected under most Good amaritan laws if they perform CPR, even if they have had no formal training. iood Samaritan laws have been expanded in a number of jurisdictions to rotect from liability laypersons and health professionals who do not have a duty) respond, who are acting "in good faith" and are not guilty of gross negligence.

laving gone to the aid of an injured diver, a rescuer must administer the ssistance with reasonable care. Thus, for example, before commencing CPR, ie rescuer should check the injured diver's airway, breathing and circulation, eing aware of the risks of performing resuscitation techniques on a person who oes not require it. When administering CPR (or any other first aid procedure), escuers must do so according to their level of training and experience.

he reasonably prudent CPR provider would not arbitrarily abandon the injured liver or cease resuscitation without a valid reason (eg. relieved by another qualified person who takes over resuscitation efforts, or exhaustion of the escuer). Ethically and legally there is no distinction between continuing CPR ind not starting it in the first place, as long as it is required.

he rescuer is not expected to work miracles, and a court is unlikely to require a escuer to ensure the survival of the injured diver. Given that the injured diver is utside hospital, is not breathing, has no pulse and is probably, or will shortly be, :linically dead, all that is required of the rescuer is a genuine attempt to revive he diver by the exercise of common sense and an appropriate and reasonable Jegree of skill.

It is most unlikely that an injured diver who, but for the timely intervention of the rescuer would be dead, would succeed in recovering damages for broken ribs or internal injury caused by appropriate external chest compressions. Legal action is far more likely to be initiated and succeed where the injured diver was breathing and/or clearly had a pulse, but was further injured or died as a consequence of inappropriate CPR administration. Conceivably, the dependants of a victim who was not successfully resuscitated might sue the rescuer for damages.

Any action, whether brought by the injured diver or by the dependants of a victim, would be based upon an allegation of negligence, or more precisely, the breach of a duty owed by the rescuer to the injured diver. The claimant must establish not only the existence of such a duty of care, but a breach of that duty and some injury or loss that was so caused.

In the sort of emergency situation contemplated, where a first aider comes upon a clinically dead diver, it is most unlikely the dependants would succeed in establishing that the death of a victim was caused by the efforts of the first aider. The first aider cannot be held accountable for the injured diver's medical condition prior to commencing CPR, and, if attempts at resuscitation fail, the diver's clinical status was not worsened from when discovered with no pulse, in a non-breathing and clinically dead state.

In his article in *Alert Diver* 1 (2) 1995, Lawrence Shindell reports that although there are few reported cases construing Good Samaritan laws, courts in three states have denied protection under broadly written Good Samaritan statutes applying to "anyone" rendering first aid, based on the existance of a pre-existing duty arising from a relationship of some form. None of these cases involved recreational scuba divers or diving professionals.

Divemasters and Instructors

The training of a divemaster or instructor usually incorporates a component of CPR with first aid. In the event of an accident involving a diver for whom the divemaster or instructor is responsible, it is likely that provision of assistance would be expected, unlike the case of a stranger. The divemaster or instructor could then be expected to demonstrate a reasonable proficiency in the rescue and provision of first aid consistent with the level of training.

In addition, where a term of the contract between an instructor and a student requires it, the instructor may have a contractual obligation to assist.

OXYGEN FIRST AID

Although it is generally regarded as safe to provide oxygen to a diver thought to be suffering from a diving-related injury, there has been some concern about the possible legal ramifications of doing so.

In the United States, the first aid provider must obtain permission from an injured person prior to administering first aid. This means that the oxygen provider must obtain permission from the injured diver before providing oxygen. The Divers Alert Network has suggested that the oxygen provider say something like: *"This is oxygen. It may make you feel better. May I help you?"* This is consistent with first aid standard of practice for obtaining informed consent. For unconscious injured divers, permission is assumed.

The Food and Drug Administration (FDA) regulates oxygen as a therapy drug. A prescription from a licensed physician is required for its purchase and use. However, this requirement has never been enforced for the use of oxygen in emergency situations. Although a proposed ruling was made by the FDA to remove the prescription requirement from oxygen in 1972, it was never implemented. The "Use Statement" in the 1972 Federal Register, 37 (52) reads: "For oxygen deficiency or emergency resuscitation when used by personnel properly instructed in oxygen administration. For other medical applications only as directed by a physician." This statement appears to permit qualified laypersons to obtain and provide oxygen in emergency situations without a prescription.

The FDA is currently reviewing its position on this matter. In the interim, it appears that the 1972 Federal Register notification is being followed. DAN is deeply involved in the review process and oxygen providers should monitor *Alert Diver* for progress reports.

Some states have regulations regarding oxygen usage and a potential oxygen provider should be aware of pertinent regulations in the state(s) where they may need to provide oxygen.

In the Final Summary of Recommendations from the 1990 Undersea and Hyperbaric Medical Society (UHMS) Diving Accident Workshop, it is stated: "... It is further suggested that dive instructors and divemasters who are responsible for conducting dives be trained in the use of oxygen. The absence of an individual trained in oxygen administration should not preclude equipping a given dive boat with oxygen apparatus ..."

First aiders are normally safe from litigation as long as they deliver first aid within their levels of training. However, a first aider who goes beyond their level of training may create a potentially dangerous situation for an injured diver and may expose themself to the threat of legal liability for causing the injury or death of the casualty.

For example, if a person, untrained in the use of a positive pressure oxygen resuscitator, attempted to resuscitate an injured diver using such a device and caused the diver to regurgitate, aspirate stomach contents and consequently die, then that person may be held responsible at law. However, some experts argue that the side effects of oxygen are so minimal that one should not withhold it from a *spontaneously breathing diver* merely because of fear of doing harm. The 1992 CPR guidelines of the American Heart Association state, in part: "... oxygen should not be withheld for fear of suppressing respiration if hypoxemia is suspected or if significant respiratory distress is present. The rescuer should be prepared to provide assisted ventilation if necessary."

Bearing in mind the UHMS statement, any dive operator should provide oxygen equipment. Every divemaster and instructor should be trained in and practised with the provision of oxygen both to breathing and non-breathing divers. Anything less than this may be regarded by a court as a departure from the appropriate duty of care.

It has often been acknowledged that regular retraining and practice are required to maintain proficiency in resuscitation techniques. First aiders should ensure that their qualifications are current.

A court is most unlikely to require a rescuer to imperil personal safety or risk life in the course of providing rescue or first aid. Thus, first aid may be administered only so long as rescuers are physically and mentally able to do so without injuring or harming themselves. If a question of possible cross infection (eg. HI hepatitis B, hepatitis C) arises, a rescuer would not be expected to jeopardia personal health.

The American Heart Association has stated: "The layperson who responds to a emergency in an unknown victim should be guided by the moral and ethica values of preserving life and assisting those in distress, balanced against th risk that may exist in the various rescue situations." (JAMA, 1992) However, goes on to say ... "If a lone rescuer refuses to initiate mouth-to-mouth ventilation he or she should at least access the EMS system, open the airway, and perforr chest compressions until a rescuer arrives who is willing to provide ventilation c until ventilation can be initiated by skilled rescuers (arriving EMTs c paramedics) with the necessary barrier devices.

APPENDICES

GLOSSARY

Abdomen: The part of the body between the chest and the pelvis.

Airway: The passages through which the air passes from the atmosphere through the nose and/or mouth to the lungs.

Angle of the jaw: The sharp bend in the lower jaw just below the ears.

Bag-valve-mask resuscitator: A resuscitation device incorporating a self-inflating bag attached to directional valves and a tight-sealing mask.

Cardiac arrest: Inability of the heart to expel its contents and generate effective circulation. It is confirmed by the absence of the carotid pulse in an unconscious, non-breathing person.

Cardiopulmonary resuscitation (CPR): Application of a combination of rescue breathing and external chest compressions to provide oxygenation and circulation to a pulseless person.

Carotid pulse: The pulse of the carotid arteries, found on each side of the neck.

Central nervous system (CNS) oxygen toxicity: Toxic effect on the brain caused by breathing oxygen concentrations usually greater than 1.6 ATA.

Chin lift: Supporting the jaw at the point of the chin in such a way that there is no pressure on the soft tissues of the neck.

Circulation: Blood flow through the heart and blood vessels to provide oxygen and nutrients to the body tissues.

Constant flow delivery system: A system that provides a constant flow of oxygen at either a fixed or adjustable flow rate.

Controlled ventilation: A term sometimes used to describe the situation when a first aider is ventilating a non-breathing person.

Cyanosis: Blueness of the skin and lining of the mouth, generally caused by lack of oxygen in the blood.

Defibrillator: Electrical device used to stop ventricular fibrillation and restore normal heart rhythm.

Demand system: A system that delivers a flow of gas when triggered by the inhalation of a spontaneously breathing person.

Expired air resuscitation (EAR): See Rescue breathing.

External chest compression (ECC): Technique applied to a pulseless person during which the lower sternum is rythmically compressed to provide circulation.

Head tilt: Backward tilting of the head on the neck.

Heimlich maneuver: Subdiaphragmatic abdominal thrusts used to clear a blocked airway.

Hemoglobin: The oxygen-carrying red-colored, iron-based compound of the red blood cells.

Hyperventilation: Overbreathing. Results in reduced blood carbon dioxide levels and reduced respiratory drive.

Hypoxemia: Below normal oxygenation of the blood.

Hypoxia: A condition in which there is less than the normal content of oxygen in the body tissues.

Inflation: The movement of gas to the injured person's lungs by means of a first aider's expired air or the use of resuscitation equipment.

Jaw support: Supporting the jaw by means of chin lift or jaw thrust.

Jaw thrust: The forward pressure applied behind the angle of the jaw to thrust the jaw forward and open the airway.

Laryngospasm (Laryngeal spasm): Persisting spasm of the muscles of the larynx resulting in partial or complete blockage to the entrance of the trachea. Usually caused by irritation from a foreign body, mucus or vomit.

Larynx: A passageway connecting the pharynx and trachea (windpipe). It is composed of plates of firm cartilage which support the vocal cords.

Manikin: A model of the human body, or the head and torso, used for resuscitation training.

Manually triggered oxygen-powered resuscitator: A resuscitation device utilizing a manual trigger or button to activate the flow of oxygen used to inflate the lungs of a non-breathing person.

Oxygen resuscitation: Ventilating a non-breathing person using elevated oxygen concentrations.

Oxygen provision: The provision of elevated inspired oxygen concentrations to an injured person.

Partial pressure: The partial pressure of a gas in a gas mixture is that part of the total pressure of the mixture that is contributed by that gas.

Perfusion: Blood supply.

Pharynx: The throat.

Positive pressure ventilation: Inflating a non-breathing person's lungs by means of pressure generated by the expired breath of the first aider or resuscitation equipment.

Pulmonary oxygen toxicity: Toxic effect on the lungs caused by breathing oxygen concentrations greater than about 0.6 ATA for extended periods.

Regurgitation: The passive outflow of stomach contents, often caused by gas entering the stomach during positive pressure ventilation. Occurs without obvious muscular action.

Rescue breathing: Involves a first aider using their expired breath to inflate the lungs and ventilate a non-breathing person. Sometimes known as expired air resuscitation or mouth-to-mouth resuscitation.

Respiration (Ventilation, Breathing): Spontaneous movement of gases in and out of the lungs.

Respiratory minute volume: The amount of gas breathed in or out during one minute. It is the tidal volume multiplied by the respiratory rate.

Resuscitation: The preservation or restoration of life by the establishment and/or maintenance of the airway, breathing and circulation - A.B.C.- and related emergency care.

Safety/pressure relief valve: Pressure limiting valve set to open at a pre-determined pressure to protect the equipment or the injured person.

Shock: Shock occurs when the circulation is inadequate to meet the oxygen demands of the major body organs.

Sternum: Breastbone, situated in the middle of the front of the chest.

Tidal volume: This is the volume of gas that moves in or out of the lungs with each breath.

Unconsciousness: For the purposes of this book, unconsciousness is defined as the condition in which an injured person fails to respond to the spoken word, obey a shouted command, or respond to the firm touch of a potential rescuer.

Ventilation: The movement of gas to the injured person's lungs by means of a first aider's expired air or the use of resuscitation equipment.

Ventricular fibrillation: Uncoordinated and irregular contraction of the heart muscles so that tremors occur and no effective circulation is generated.

Vomiting: Forceful ejection of stomach contents through the mouth by violent contraction of the muscles of the small intestine and stomach.

Xiphoid process: A knob of cartilage attached to the lowest part of the sternum.

BIBLIOGRAPHY

Acott C. Oxygen Therapy. Skindiving 1985; 16 (1): 22-26.

Acott C. First Aid Oxygen Therapy. Scuba Diver 1991; Dec/Jan: 45-49.

Agar J. Regulators used with pure oxygen. Engineering Bulletin No. 137, Airdive Equipment P/L, 1986.

Anderson D, Nagasawa G et al. O_2 pressures between 0.12 and 2.5 atm abs, circulatory function, and N_2 elimination. Undersea Biomed Res 1991; 18(4): 279-292.

Australian Resuscitation Council Policy Statement Manual. Melbourne: Australian Resuscitation Council, 1991.

Bennett PB and Elliott DH (eds). The Physiology and Medicine of Diving (3rd Edn). San Pedro: Best Publishing Co, 1982.

Bennett PB and Moon RE (eds). Diving Accident Management. UHMS Publication #78(DIVACC)12/1/90. Bethesda: Undersea and Hyperbaric Medical Society, 1990.

Betts J. Oxygen Onus. Diver 1985; 30 (10): 11.

Bove AA and Davis JC. Diving Medicine (2nd Edn). Philadelphia: W.B. Saunders Co,1990.

British Sub-Aqua Club. Safety and Rescue for Divers. London: Stanley Paul, 1987.

Cardiopulmonary Resuscitation. Melbourne: Australian Resuscitation Council, 1989.

Centers for Disease Control. Guidelines for prevention of transmission of human immunodeficiency virus and hepatitis B virus to health-care and public-safety workers. MMWR 1989; 88 (suppl 6): 1-37.

Chandra N, Rudikoff M and Weisfeldt ML. Simultaneous Chest Compression and Ventilation at High Airway Pressure During Cardiopulmonary Resuscitation. Lancet 1980, 41: 175-178.

Clark J. Oxygen Poisoning. In: Davis JC (ed), Hyperbaric and Undersea Medicine. California: Medical Seminars Inc, 1981.

Clark J. Oxygen Toxicity. In: Bennett PB and Elliott DH (eds), The Physiology and Medicine of Diving (3rd Edn). California: Best Publishing Co, 1982: 200-238.

Corry JA. Oxygen's Role in Dive Accident Management. NDA News 1985; Nov/Dec: 31.

Corry JA. Diver Rescue Management. Proceedings of the Diving Officers' Conference. London: BS-AC, 1986.

Corry JA. Student Workbook for Emergency Oxygen Administration Workshop. Montclair: NAUI, 1987.

Corry JA. Setting the record straight: Oxygen delivery and the injured diver. In Bennett, PB and Moon, RE (eds). Diving Accident Management. UHMS Publication #78(DIVACC)12/1/90. Bethesda: Undersea and Hyperbaric Medical Society, 1990.

Davies T. Oxygen to the Rescue. Diver 1986; 31 (5): 16-17.

Davis JC and Youngblood D. Definitive Treatment of Decompression Sickness and Arterial Gas Embolism. In: Davis JC (ed). Hyperbaric and Undersea Medicine. California: Medical Seminars Inc, 1981.

Davis JC. Hyperbaric Oxygen Therapy: Applications in Clinical Practice. In: Davis JC (ed). Hyperbaric and Undersea Medicine. California: Medical Seminars Inc, 1981.

Davis JC and Elliott DH. Treatment of the Decompression Disorders. In: Bennett PB and Elliott DH (eds). The Physiology and Medicine of Diving (3rd Edn). San Pedro: Best Publishing Co, 1982: 473-487.

Dick A, Bennett PB and Miller JN. Oxygen and Diving Accidents. Alert Diver 1985; 2 (1): 1-2.

Disease Transmission Concerns in Diver and CPR Training. In: The Undersea Journal 1987; Third Quarter: 42-43.

Divers Alert Network. 1988 Report. North Carolina: Divers Alert Network, 1988.

Divers Alert Network. Report on 1988 Diving Accidents. Durham: Divers Alert Network, 1989.

Divers Alert Network. 1989 Report on Diving Accidents and Fatalities. Durham: Divers Alert Network, 1991.

Divers Alert Network. 1991 Underwater Diving Accident Manual. Durham, Divers Alert Network, 1991.

Donald K. Oxygen and the Diver. Worcs: The SPA Ltd, 1992.

Dueker CW. Scuba Diving in Safety and Health. Menlo Park: Diving Safety Digest, 1985.

Dovenbarger J. Oxygen Use in Dive Accidents. Alert Diver 1988; 4 (2): 12-13.

Duncan J. A Legal Perspective. In: Diving Accident Management in Australia. Sydney: PADI Australia, 1988.

Edmonds C, Lowry C and Pennefather J. Diving and Subaquatic Medicine (3rd Edn). London: Butterworth-Heinemann Ltd, 1992.

Edmonds C, Mc Kenzie B and Thomas R. Diving Medicine for Scuba Divers. Melbourne: J.L. Publications, 1992.

Elling R and Politis J. An Evaluation of Emergency Medical Technicians' Ability to Use Manual Ventilation Devices. Annals of Emergency Medicine 1983; 12: 765-768.

Gardener JF and Peel MM. Introduction to sterilization and disinfection (2nd Edn). Melbourne: Churchill Livingston, 1991.

Gatehouse M and Wodak T. The Diving Instructor and The Law. FAUI News 1988; 10 (1): 12-14.

Grant HD et al. Emergency Care (4th Edn). New Jersey: Brady, 1989.

Guidelines for Cardiopulmonary Resuscitation and Emergency Cardiac Care. In: The Journal of The American Medical Association (JAMA); 1992; 268 (16): 2172-2299.

Harnett R et al. A Review of the Literature Concerning Resuscitation from Hypothermia: Part 1 - The Problem and General Approaches. Aviat Space and Environ Med 1983; 54 (5): 425-434.

Harnett R et al. A Review of the Literature Concerning Resuscitation from Hypothermia: Part 11 - Selected Rewarming Protocols. Aviat Space and Environ Med 1983; 54 (6): 487-495.

Hendrick W and Thomson B. Oxygen and the Scuba Diver. New York: Lifeguard Systems Inc, 1988.

Hyldegaard O, Moller M and Madsen J. Effect of He-O_2, O_2 and N_2O-O_2 breathing on injected bubbles in spinal white matter. Undersea Biomed Res 1991; 18 (5 & 6): 361-371.

Johannigman JA and Branson RD. Oxygen Enrichment of Expired Gas for Mouth-to-Mask Resuscitation. Respiratory Care 1991; 36 (2): 99-103.

Komesaroff D. The Use of Bi-Nasal Oxygen Cannulae in Expired Air Resuscitation. Technical Committee Research Project. Melbourne: The Royal Life Saving Society of Australia, 1980.

Komesaroff D. Cardiopulmonary Resuscitation. Melbourne: Victorian Academy for General Practice Ltd, 1982.

Lawrence PJ and Sivaneswaran N. Ventilation during cardiopulmonary resuscitation: which method? The Medical Journal of Australia 1985; 143: 443-446.

Leigh JM. Variation in performance of oxygen therapy devices. Anaesthesia 1970; 25 (2): 210-222.

Lippmann J. Deeper Into Diving. Melbourne: J.L. Publications, 1990.

Lippmann J and Bugg S. The DAN Emergency Handbook (2nd Edn). Melbourne: J.L. Publications, 1991.

Luce JM et al. New Developments in Cardiopulmonary Resuscitation. JAMA 1980; 244 (12): 1365-1370.

Macdonald L and Verhoeven A (eds). Australian First Aid (2nd Edn). Canberra: St John Ambulance Australia, 1990.

Maier GW et al. The physiology of external cardiac massage: high-impulse cardiopulmonary resuscitation. Circulation 1984; 70 (1): 86-101.

Montgomery WH and Herrin TJ (eds). Student Manual for Basic Life Support - Cardiopulmonary Resuscitation. Dallas: American Heart Association, 1981.

Niemann JT. Cardiopulmonary Resuscitation. The New England Journal of Medicine 1992; 327 (15): 1075-1080.

Older P. Cardiopulmonary resuscitation in hospital. Medical Journal of Australia 1985; 143: 431-432.

Page JO. CPR and the Law. The Undersea Journal 1987; Third Quarter: 19-20.

Pearn J. The Management of Near Drowning. The Journal of the Royal Life Saving Society 1991; 7: 5-10.

Petersen GM. Application and Assessment of Oxygen Therapy Devices. Nursing Clinics of North America 1981; 16 (2): 241-257.

Pocket Mask™ - Directions for Use. Stavanger: Laerdal Medical.

Pozos R and Wittmers L (eds). The Nature and Treatment of Hypothermia (Vol 2). Minneapolis: University of Minnesota Press, 1983.

Resuscitation and Emergency Care. Sydney: The Royal Life Saving Society - Australia, 1987.

Rhoades R and Pflanzer R. Human Physiology. Philadelphia: Saunders College Publishers, 1989.

Rudikoff MT et al. Mechanisms of Blood Flow During Cardiopulmonary Resuscitation. Circulation 1980; 61 (2): 345-352.

Rutala WA. APIC Guideline for Selection and Use of Disinfectants. In: American Journal of Infection Control 1990; 18 (2): 99-117.

Safar P and Bircher N. Cardiopulmonary Cerebral Resuscitation (3rd Edn). London: W.B Saunders Co Ltd, 1988

Smart DR and Mark PD. Oxygen therapy in emergency medicine. Part 1. Physiology and oxygen delivery systems. Emergency Medicine 1992; 4 (3): 163-178.

Spearing Bolgiano C et al. Administering Oxygen Therapy: What You Need to Know. Nursing 1990; June: 47-51.

Standards and Guidelines for Cardiopulmonary Resuscitation and Emergency Cardiac Care. In: The Journal of The American Medical Association (JAMA); 1986; 255 (21): 2841-3044.

Sterba JA. Field Management of Accidental Hypothermia During Diving. In: Bennett, PB and Moon, RE (eds). Diving Accident Management. UHMS

Publication #78(DIVACC)12/1/90. Bethesda: Undersea and Hyperbaric Medical Society, 1990.

Stewart AG and Howard P. Devices for low flow O_2 administration. Eur Respir J 1990; 3: 812-817.

Swenson RD et al. Hemodynamics in Humans During Conventional and Experimental Methods of Cardiopulmonary Resuscitation. Circulation 1988; 78: 630-639.

Taylor L. Rx: Oxygen - The Legal Issues. Alert Diver 1986; 2 (5): 10.

Taylor L. A Diver's Guide to Oxygen Therapy - Part 1. Sources 1989; 1 (2): 30-35.

Taylor L. A Diver's Guide to Oxygen Therapy - Part 2. Sources 1989; 1 (3): 72-74.

Taylor L. A Higher Concentration Oxygen Delivery Pocket Mask, Alert Diver 1989, 5 (3): 15.

Tortora G and Anagnostakos N. Principles of Anatomy and Physiology (5th Edn). New York: Harper and Row, 1987.

Vander A et al. Human Physiology: The Mechanisms of Body Function. Sydney: McGraw-Hill, 1985.

Walters D. Oxygen - Friend or foe? Skindiving 1985; April/May: 85-86.

Work K. MedDive. Colorado: Dive Rescue Inc, 1991.

ANSWERS TO EXERCISES

Chapter 1

1. Arteries have thick, elastic walls that resist stretching, thereby maintaining the blood pressure. Most arteries carry oxygenated blood. Veins are often larger, and are thin-walled, directing the blood flow by means of one-way valves. Most veins carry deoxygenated blood.

2. Plasma - carries sugar, other nutritional compounds and various other substances; red cells - carry hemoglobin, which bonds with oxygen, allowing it to be transported through the body; white cells - fight bacterial infection; and platelets - activate clotting.

3. Most is chemically combined with hemoglobin. A relatively small proportion is dissolved in plasma.

4. Passage of a gas from an area where it has a high concentration to an area where its concentration is lower, until the concentrations are equal.

5. Major trigger provided by chemoreceptors in the medulla which detect rising blood carbon dioxide levels. Other receptors in the carotid arteries and aorta may activate breathing if blood oxygen levels become dangerously low.

6. Drowsiness, incoordination, headache, double vision, possible euphoria, apathy, blueness of lips, mouth and fingernail beds, rapid pulse and breathing, convulsions, unconsciousness and death.

7. Rapid, deep breathing, shortness of breath, throbbing headache, dizziness, nausea, confusion, unsteadiness, disorientation, restlessness, flushed warm face, lightheadedness, muscle twitches and jerks, reduced vision, unconsiousness, tremors, convulsions, death.

8. 500 ml for a 150 pound adult at rest.

Chapter 2

1. Reduction in effective circulation resulting in an inadequate supply of oxygen to vital organs.

2. Signs and symptoms of shock include: cold clammy pale skin, rapid weak pulse, rapid shallow breathing, weakness, thirst, nausea, vomiting and apprehension.

3. First aid for shock includes: monitoring of vital signs and resuscitation if necessary; determining the cause and acting to rectify it; stopping severe external bleeding; laying the diver down; oxygen provision; arranging medical assistance or advice; keeping the diver still, quiet and reassured and recording details of the accident and injured diver's condition and treatment.

4. If the cause of shock is not rectified the injured diver may deteriorate rapidly. Many first aiders lack adequate experience to determine whether further treatment will be required.

Chapter 3

1. Death of brain tissue usually begins after about 3-5 minutes of oxygen deprivation.

2. Might have a spinal injury which can be easily aggravated.

3. Head tilt and chin lift, or jaw thrust if spinal injury is suspected.

4. If an unconscious diver is left lying on the back, the lower jaw drops and the tongue, which is attached to the jaw, drops back against the back of the throat, partly or completely blocking the passage of air to the lungs.

5. In case they vomit, to drain fluids, and help keep the airway open.

6. Where the emergency is, the telephone number from which the call is made, the nature of the problem, how many divers need help, the condition of the diver(s) and what aid is being administered.

7. Just hard enough to cause the lower chest and abdomen to rise.

8. Reduces the chance of gastric distension. In addition, during controlled ventilation, better gas exchange occurs during expiration when the pressure is relieved and the pulmonary capillaries are well perfused.

9. Carotid pulse for 5-10 seconds.

10. Scoop visible foreign matter from the mouth. Try subdiaphragmatic abdominal thrusts. If this fails, finger sweeps are tried. The sequence is repeated as necessary.

11. Blowing too hard, not allowing the chest to fall before ventilating again, inadequately opened or clear airway, pressure on the stomach.

12. Regurgitation is passive. Vomiting is accompanied by active muscular spasm.

13. Clear airway, maximum head tilt/chin lift, do not overventilate and ensure the chest falls before ventilating again.

14. No detectable carotid pulse.

15. 2 breaths and 15 compressions with a compression rate of 80-100 per minute.

16. 1 breath and 5 compressions with a compression rate of 80-100 per minute.

17. Color of injured diver's lips and skin and maintenance of spontaneous pulse.

18. Improvement in the color of the injured diver, the presence of an artificial pulse (2 rescuers) and return of a spontaneous pulse.

Chapter 4

1. Extreme fatigue, numbness, tingling, headache, joint pain, other body pain, weakness, vision or speech difficulty, decreased consciousness, incoordination, paralysis.

2. Adds no more nitrogen, washes out dissolved nitrogen, washes out the nitrogen in bubbles thus reducing bubble size, improves tissue oxygenation, reduces respiratory distress, reduces shock, cerebral edema, blood sludging.

3. Chest pain, shortness of breath, coughing, cyanosis and shock.

4. Reduces hypoxia by increasing diffusion of oxygen across damaged or poorly perfused lung surface. Reduces size of pneumothoraces and mediastinal air by nitrogen elimination.

5. Helps break the bond between carbon monoxide and hemoglobin and other tissue proteins. Increases amount of oxygen dissolved in plasma.

Chapter 5

1. Horizontally without the head or legs elevated.

2. As soon as possible after an accident to gain the maximum benefit.

3. Until the supply is depleted or advised by a physician to cease oxygen provision.

4. Temporarily if the diver vomits, regurgitates, during a seizure, or when the supply is depleted.

5. The underlying cause of the problem may still be present although the symptoms have abated.

Chapter 6

1. About 18-48 hours.

2. By giving air breaks for 5 minutes after every 25 minutes on 100% oxygen.

3. Usually 1.6 ATA but has occurred at lower pressures.

4. The diver's rapid demands for breath may not easily be met due to the breathing resistance of the demand valve. This may increase the anxiety and magnify the problem.

Chapter 7

1. Fire hazard from oxygen gas, potential for explosion of cylinder, endangering injured diver by improper use of certain positive pressure equipment.

2. Cannot see, smell or taste oxygen.

3. Normally every 5 years. May be extended to 10 years for steel cyllinders with a star symbol.

4. May contain harmful contaminants due to less stringent cleaning and filling procedures than those used with medical oxygen.

5. Adequate oxygen supply to allow an injured diver to breath oxygen from the dive site until reaching an appropriate medical facility or recompression chamber.

6. Approximately 2000 - 2200 psi.

7. To minimize the heat build-up and so reduce the chance of ignition, as well as to reduce the stress on the equipment caused by a very rapid pressure build-up.

8. May contain lubricants or other substances that are incompatible with high oxygen pressures.

Chapter 8

1. So the oxygen provider can see if the injured diver regurgitates or vomits, to allow observation of the person's face and lip color, and can see if spontaneous breathing is occurring by checking if the interior of the mask is temporarily fogging up after exhalation.

2. Via a demand valve delivery system.

3. There may be insufficient suction to open the valve.

4. The oxygen provider can breathe the oxygen from the demand valve (with their nose sealed) and then exhales their expired breath into the injured diver.

5. Because high flowrates are required to achieve high oxygen concentrations with constant flow systems.

6. Seal on the face, minute volume of the injured diver, shaping of clear plastic masks over the nose, oxygen flow rate and the type of delivery system,

7. If an effective seal is not achieved, it is often difficult to generate sufficent tidal volumes to adequately ventilate a non-breathing diver.

8. Such devices are easily capable of inflating the stomach and causing regurgitation. In addition, most of these devices have the potential to generate enough pressure to cause pulmonary barotrauma.

9. Exhaustion of soda lime could cause carbon dioxide toxicity. Slight possibility of inhaling soda lime dust. Difficult for an operator to ventilate a non-breathing person unless they are highly skilled.

Chapter 9

1. By using the demand inhalator valve with the Tru Fit™ or Pocket Mask™ attached.

2. The non-rebreather mask attached to the barbed flow outlet.

3. A minimum flow rate of 15 lpm.

4. By performing rescue breathing using the Pocket Mask™ attached to the barbed outlet, and with a minimum oxygen flow rate of 15 lpm.

Chapter 10

1. To aspirate fluid matter such as water, mucus, saliva and vomit from the mouth and nose, thereby preventing inhalation of the fluids and helping clear the airway.

2. No further than the back teeth. If a diver is not deeply unconscious, placing a suction catheter further into the throat may cause gagging or vomiting and the associated complications.

3. If left in one place, it can dry up and block on mucous membrane.

4. The oxygen supply (if required) is turned on, the lid of the collection bottle is tight, there is a seal inside the lid of the bottle and that it is in good condition, there are no cracks in the bottle or kinks or cracks in the tubing.

5. Oropharyngeal airways must only be used by those who are trained to use them.

6. They prevent airway obstruction by the tongue, lips and teeth.

7. If inserted in a conscious or semi-conscious diver whose upper airway reflexes are intact, an oropharyngeal airway can cause vomiting or laryngospasm.

Chapter 11

1. To prevent moisture and other contaminants from entering.

2. Relieves the pressure on valve seats and various other parts and increases their lifetime.

3. So they can be quickly unpacked and used effectively when required.

4. Any build-up of oxygen could cause a fire.

Chapter 12

1. Blood.

2. Disposable rubber gloves, towels etc and resuscitation masks.

3. As soon as possible after use.

4. Disposable parts are discarded. The equipment is disassembled, appropriate parts are pre-rinsed with cold, running water and then washed thoroughly in warm water using a detergent that is compatible with the resuscitator materials. The parts are then rinsed thoroughly in clean water prior to sterilization.

5. The parts are rinsed thoroughly in clean water, dried, and the equipment is reassembled and tested.

DAN OXYGEN COURSE AND MEMBERSHIP INFORMATION

The DAN *Oxygen First Aid in Dive Accidents* course was designed to fill the void in oxygen first aid training available for the general diving public.

Course Description

This course represents entry level training designed to educate the general diving (and qualified non-diving) public in recognizing possible dive-related injuries; and providing emergency oxygen first aid while activating the local emergency medical services (EMS) and/or arranging for evacuation to the nearest available medical facility.

Course Highlights

- Introduction/Overview
- Course Objectives
- Physiology Review
- Recognition of Dive Accidents
- Review of Dive Emergencies
- Overview of Dive Accident Statistics

- Benefits of Oxygen
- Introduction to Oxygen Equipment
- Skills Practice and Mastery
- Final Examination
- Review with discussion
- Certification

Course Prerequisites

- CPR training from a nationally recognized agency.
- DAN Membership strongly recommended.
- Junior diver certified participants are advised to be accompanied by their adult buddy.

Course Objectives

- Recognize signs and symptoms of a dive emergency requiring oxygen first aid.
- State the benefits of providing oxygen to an injured diver.
- State potential hazards of working with oxygen.
- Assemble and deploy the DAN Oxygen Unit with skill and confidence.
- State the circumstances under which each mask option (demand, non-rebreather and pocket) is used for breathing and non-breathing injured divers.

For more information, contact DAN Training Division at (919) 684-2948 extension 555.

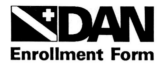

Enrollment Form

For quick enrollment call 1-800-446-2671

Name(s)

_____

_____

Address

_____

_____

Day Phone (   ) _____

Current DAN Member   No   Yes

Member Number _____

I am enclosing:

☐ **$25 for DAN Membership** $ _____

☐ **$35 for DAN Family Membership** $ _____

☐ **For $15,000 medical insurance, add $20 per person** $ _____

☐ **For $30,000 medical insurance, add $25 per person** $ _____

          Total Enclosed **$** _____

Only residents of U.S. and Canada are eligible for insurance. Please include an additional $5 if outside U.S.

Type of payment please circle:

Check/Money Order VISA MasterCard

Card # _____

Expiration Date _____

Signature _____

Date _____

*Please return application to: **DAN**, Box 3823, Duke University Medical Center, Durham, North Carolina 27710 or call **1-800-446-2671** or **(919) 684-2948**.*

INDEX

OTHER BOOKS BY JOHN LIPPMANN

The DAN Emergency Handbook (2nd Edn) by John Lippmann and Stan Bugg. Melbourne: J.L. Publications, 1991.

A guide to the identification of and first aid for SCUBA diving injuries. An essential reference for all divers.

Deeper Into Diving by John Lippmann. Melbourne: J.L. Publications, 1990.

A very detailed technical review of most of the available decompression procedures and the physical and physiological aspects of deeper diving. An essential reference for divemasters, instructors and other diving professionals.

The Essentials of Deeper (Sport) Diving by John Lippmann. New York: Aqua Quest Publications Inc, 1992.

An overview of the theory and requirements of deeper diving. Very interesting and useful reading for all divers.

For advice on diving-related illnesses, telephone DAN on:

919-684-8111 diving emergency (24 hours)

919-684-2948 information only
